Conquer Fatigue

*A Wellness Program to Increase
Your Energy, Vitality & Productivity*

In 30 Days

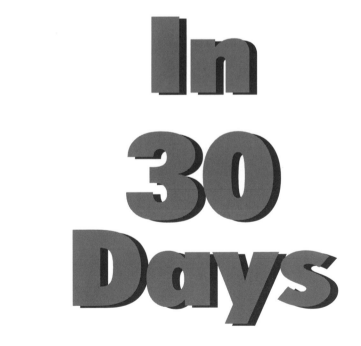

By Dr. Elizabeth Walker

Conquer Fatigue in 30 Days

Published by Vitality Doctor
1700 South College Ave, Suite C, Fort Collins, Colorado 80525

Walker, Elizabeth
      Conquer Fatigue in 30 Days / Dr. Elizabeth Walker
      Fort Collins, CO: Vitality Doctor
            Includes bibliographical references and index.
            ISBN 0-9704348-0-4
            1. Health and Fitness 2. Medical 3. Nutrition
            4. Chronic Fatigue Syndrome 5. Self-help I. Title

Printed in the United States of America
1-10

This book is dedicated to my son Ryan,
God's gift to boost my hope and faith
to understand that beyond all suffering
lies some of life's greatest treasures.

Acknowledgements

I wish to thank the following people for inspiring my health career and assisting me on the journey of wellness, vitality and longevity:

Jack LaLanne, Emmanuel Cheraskin, M.D., D.M.D., Joseph Lipari, D.C., The National College of Chiropractic, Raymond Bayley, D.C., David and Cindy Briscoe, Jan Ste. Germaine, M.S., Larry Herbig, D.C., Walter Schmitt, D.C., DACBN, Michael Lebowitz, D.C., Jeffrey Bland, Ph.D., Jeff and Michael Katke, Lyra Heller, M.A., Brad Rachman, D.C., and Mark Percival, D.C., N. D.

My sincerest thanks and appreciation to the following people for their help on this book:

- My wonderful assistant, Charis Gregory, for her editing, internet research, charts and graphs, and managing the office so I could put my time and attention into writing this book
- Gretchen Gaede, of The Write Words, for her excellent editing, formatting, layout and indexing skills and bringing the whole project together
- Tara Jensen of Silver Lining Enterprises for the front cover digital photography and exercise photography for *Day 28- How's Your Posture?*
- Kelly Breeden of Color Key for the cover design, along with Donna Murphy, who also helped with editing
- Betsy Strafach of Portraits by Betsy for the back cover photograph
- Dr. Larry Herbig, for his helpful editing and input on several key chapters
- Jan Ste. Germaine, M.S., Diplomate in Acupuncture, Chinese Herbology and Oriental Medicine; for her suggestions on chapters
- My sister, Janet Johnson, and friends, Dr. Terry Spencer and Cindy Boyle for their encouragement and support throughout this project and for many years during my illness
- My son, Ryan, who inspires me to be the best I can be
- My parents, Ben and Beryl Eppele, who have guided this project from heaven
- Susan Geiser, for her helpful editing

I wish to thank the following people for their guidance to my career as a speaker and author:

Jack Canfield, Mark Victor Hansen, Jerrold R. Jenkins, Tony Robbins, Dottie Walters and my many friends and mentors in the National Speakers Association.

> **"What you are is God's gift to you.
> What you make of yourself is your gift to God."**
> **--Anonymous**

I have had a plaque with that quote for probably 30 years. It got me through the "Me Decade" of the eighties. Even though this is a "self help" book, its true purpose is to help you achieve your body's full potential so you can fulfill your life's mission and be a blessing to others. If you are weak, sick or tired, you are not going to have any energy left for anyone other than yourself. It is my deepest wish that you become strong, energetic and powerful and show the world what you are made of!

A NOTE TO READERS

This book is not intended to replace the advice and treatment of a physician. Any use of the information set forth herein is entirely at the reader's discretion. The author and publisher advise that a person using this manual have the medical tests necessary to rule out or identify serious disease. If you are presently undergoing treatment for some condition and want to use this manual to augment those methods please discuss this with your doctor or licensed health professional.

Because every person's health is different, there is always some risk involved in self-treatment. Please do not use this book if you are unwilling to assume that risk. The author and publisher are not responsible for any adverse effects or consequences resulting from the use of any information, products, preparations or procedures described in this book.

Table of Contents

Preface

Cherish Your Health

The first several years of my practice were extremely frustrating. Here I was, an authority on healing and *I could not even heal myself!* My illness began twenty years ago, in my first year of chiropractic college. It was a bizarre autoimmune disorder with severe, daily hives and itching, fatigue, insomnia, food allergies and multiple chemical sensitivities, among other things.

Eventually, I realized two things: first, some of the best doctors in every profession could not heal me either; second, despite my disease, I was really much healthier than the majority of patients who came to see me. I no longer caught colds, despite frequent infections in my first twenty-two years. And if I did get sick, I was usually well enough to work, and recovered within forty-eight hours.

I came to understand I had much to offer my patients, despite my own imperfect health. My quest for healing helped me discover what worked and what did not. Other patients who were also given no hope for a cure began to find their way to my office. I discovered that restoring energy and vitality was the highest priority for those with chronic health problems. We can accept the fact that our health may never be perfect again as long as we can achieve a higher quality of life. After relocating to Colorado, I named my new office, "Vitality Doctor." My practice is dedicated to helping people regain their highest levels of energy, vitality and productivity, no matter what their diagnosis.

Having a chronic illness for twenty years forces one to examine stresses in every aspect of his or her life. My healing journey and the reversal of ninety-five percent of my symptoms, especially fatigue, are the basis for this book. There is nothing in this book I have not personally experienced. I "walk my talk" but like most people, consistently strive to do better.

One of my most important jobs as a doctor is that of a teacher. I help my clients understand what has caused their problems and how we can facilitate the body to heal itself. That's right – heal itself. When your hand is cut, you know it will usually heal without any outside assistance. The same healing force can heal more difficult health problems.

Symptoms are a sign of disharmony with health. We have to find the sources of stress and eliminate as many contributing factors as possible. This requires as much, if not more, effort on the part of the patient as on the doctor. A doctor can only help a patient to the extent of their willingness to make changes in their health habits and lifestyle.

This book provides you with information that will allow you to make better health choices. My job is that of a Health Coach. I like to tell my clients, **"*I am the steering wheel and you are the gas pedal."*** I work with each person to implement health and lifestyle changes at a different pace. There is no "one size fits all" program. All health programs require the effort of both parties to get where they want to go.

The concept of making doctors "health coaches" was initiated by **Dr. Mark Percival** of **Health Coach®️ Systems International, Inc.**, in Ontario, Canada. He has trained nearly a thousand doctors to better educate their patients on ways to take greater control over their health. Our highest purpose is to offer you compelling reasons which inspire and motivate you to choose a healthier lifestyle.

This book is designed for both individuals suffering from fatigue and their health care providers. It is my sincere desire to raise the level of knowledge about nutrition and natural healing methods among all areas of the medical field. Many doctors are frustrated by their limited knowledge of nutrition. These doctors will benefit greatly by having clear information that will enable them to better understand how to improve their patients' health and vitality.

Throughout this book I mention nutritional products by **Metagenics**, which is the number one nutritional company among doctors. The vitamin industry is vastly unregulated and the consumer has no guarantee of potency, quality, truth in labeling, pesticide contamination, germs, or heavy metals. **Metagenics** manufactures their products according to pharmacologic manufacturing practices and has their products tested for potency and quality by independent third parties. This is the evidence doctors need to get predictable results.

I choose to focus primarily on this one major company whose products I have used successfully for over fifteen years. I am not being paid by **Metagenics** to mention their products. I do not have the means to investigate the qualities of other companies and their products. I discuss specific products I use in my practice so other doctors can learn more about how to implement nutrition in their practice.

FUNCTIONAL MEDICINE

I have attended hundreds of hours of postgraduate seminars over the years and my recent focus has been training in a new branch of healing known as "Functional Medicine." This evolved from a variety of scientists, doctors and other clinicians who started to combine their collective knowledge and investigate health problems with different questions than the standard medical model. Instead of asking how to offer comfort for a particular symptom or disease, these health researchers seek to discover the cause or disrupted function that created the condition. Understanding the cause often leads to a solution that reverses the problem.

A few years ago, one of our astute mentors in this quest, **Jeffrey Bland, Ph.D**, founded the **Institute for Functional Medicine, Inc**., in Gig Harbor, Washington. This is a clinic where researchers, doctors and clinicians, of various disciplines, attempt to discover solutions to some of the body's mysteries of malfunction and disease and apply a combination of therapies from various healing arts.

His institute helps disseminate some of the best scientific, clinical knowledge available so health practitioners can digest it and put it to use in their clinics throughout the world. They offer several opportunities for physician education through seminars, on-site training and a monthly tape education series. Information on the **Institute for Functional Medicine** can be obtained by visiting their web site, **www.fxmed.com** or by calling (800) 228-0622.

CHERISH YOUR HEALTH!

"Cherish Your Health" are three words that sum up the motto of my practice and are incorporated into the logo. It is my greatest desire that everyone respect their bodies and do everything in their power to prevent disease. There is plenty of evidence to support the idea that disease prevention not only helps you live longer, but also enables you to live with fewer health problems.

Many people fear old age because they imagine themselves with chronic disease and debilitation. Growing old, however, does not have to be a time of weakness and misery. Consider someone like exercise guru, **Jack LaLanne**, who is vibrantly strong and healthy in his mid-eighties. He is an inspiration to anyone who fears aging.

> "There is no chance, no fate, no destiny
> that can circumvent, or hinder, or control
> a firm resolve of a determined soul."
> — Unknown

Introduction

Seeking the Cause

Congratulations! By purchasing this book, you have made the decision to no longer accept fatigue as "just part of getting older," or as "something you will just have to live with." Although fatigue is on the increase, this book will show you many productive ways to overcome this problem.

This book came forth as a means to put together the many concepts I have shared in my health seminars over the years. I have much more to share with you than can be conveyed or absorbed in just a few hours time. Reading this book will enable you to receive this extensive information in bite-size pieces that are more easily digested and implemented.

With each day of the thirty-day wellness program you will learn a health lesson, take a quiz or use an exercise. Hopefully, these will inspire more productive health habits to build your energy and vitality. Please resist the urge to skip over the chapters or exercises that do not appeal to you. Each step is important to help you break through barriers that are holding back your energy.

It is best not to wait until you have read the entire book to start implementing the new ideas and activities. Begin making changes, large or small, immediately! Most new tasks are designed to take only five to fifteen minutes of your day. I would encourage you to read the book a second time to reevaluate whether the changes that were initially difficult, are easier to implement the second time around.

Fatigue is the most prevalent symptom that causes someone to seek a doctor's help. It can affect you in a wide spectrum of frequency and severity. Some people have intermittent, mild symptoms, while others may have chronic or daily symptoms. At least 500,000 Americans suffer from a severe, debilitating form of fatigue known as **Chronic Fatigue Syndrome** (CFS).

There are three basic reasons for fatigue: depletion, toxicity and stress. Depletion of nutrients is very common and is often one of the easiest to correct. Toxicity unfortunately, is all too common but more difficult to alleviate. Stress is always present and can never be eliminated from our lives. However, we can change our reaction to stress through diligent efforts to change life-long unproductive or destructive habits.

Health is a choice. We have all made many choices concerning our health. We have decided whether to eat vegetarian or animal products, use tobacco, drink alcohol, and experiment with cocaine, marijuana or other illegal drugs. Understanding the consequences of our choices is the first step to making different decisions. However, knowing that something has a harmful outcome is not always a strong enough motivator. A perfect example of this is cigarette smoking.

We have known for a lifetime that smoking can have dire consequences on our health, yet it continues to be an extremely popular activity. Additionally, cigarettes are very expensive. Each pack costs an amount, which if invested properly, could enable one to take a fabulous vacation every year or add substantially to a retirement portfolio.

When I was growing up in the 50's and 60's, our families made more of a distinction between what was part of our daily diet and what was considered "party food." We only consumed soft drinks, snack foods and fancy desserts at parties. Ice cream parlors were only open during the summer months (in most Northern states). We had an abundance of family farms and home gardens, which allowed us to be much more in touch with our food and meal choices.

During my childhood, disease was much less prevalent. I never knew a child who had cancer nor even a classmate whose parent had cancer. Attention Deficit Disorders and hyperactivity were rare. We never heard of children being prescribed psychiatric drugs.

In America, the distinction between every-day diet and "party food" has blurred out of existence. Soda pop seems to have become one of the basic food groups and pop machines are now considered major "fund-raising" tools in most of our schools. School lunches have gone from hot meals or soup and sandwich to tacos, chicken fingers, fried foods, hot dogs or pizza. Ketchup is considered a vegetable. Most children will not consume breakfast cereals unless they are "frosted."

People often know the changes they should make, but do not know where to start implementing them into their lives. Strong cravings can sabotage the best intentions. Many people are convinced they will fail, so they never even begin.

In order to make this program a lifelong commitment, you have to promise yourself to practice these principles six days per week. One day of the week, allow yourself to do what you want. Party on! The day after your "party," you may experience a significant contrast from how you felt when you were following the program. This party "hangover" will give you a new perspective to help determine which of your previous habits are still important to you.

Each person has different ways of being motivated. Generally speaking, the majority of people will change in order to seek pleasure or avoid pain. The paradox is that many of the things we believe bring us pleasure are, in reality, sources of pain. This book will clarify sources of depletion, toxicity and stress and allow you to make better decisions on how to avoid pain and seek true pleasure.

Try to think beyond yourself when considering why you want to improve your energy and vitality. Other people will be impacted by your decisions. Fatigue could be the beginning of health problems that could progress into a very serious, even fatal disease. Dying a slow, painful death is not just painful to you. Think of how it will impact your loved ones.

Live each day knowing you are going to die. Quit pretending you are infallible. People who have had a close call with death often make profound changes in their life *immediately*. The best teacher is crisis. Get connected to your life purpose and live each day like it is your last.

I recently had a thirty-six-year-old friend diagnosed with colon cancer. She mentioned that she had really cleaned up her diet since the diagnosis. I asked if she would have considered changing her diet before the diagnosis if someone would have told her point blank, "Continue to eat this way and you are guaranteed to develop colon cancer." She said she probably would not have changed because of the false belief she had, like most people, we are immortal and immune to disaster.

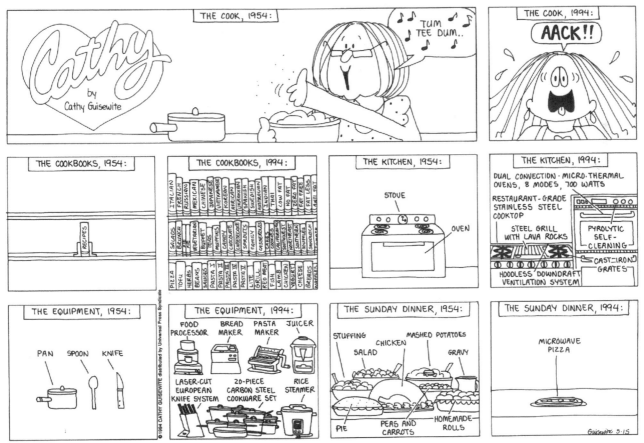

Why do we have to wait for solid evidence of a crisis? You can decide right now to make choices that greatly minimize the possibility of developing such a crisis! In my health workshops, I teach people to break out of the "victim/rescuer" model. A person who does not claim their power, or who willingly gives up their power, often makes dis-empowering choices that eventually cause them to become a victim of disease. Health is a conscious choice, not an unlimited guarantee. Resolve to be proactive, not reactive. Make a choice of how strong and healthy you want to be for the rest of your life. Your potential for good health has more to do with your actions and beliefs than your genetics.

Extensive medical detective work may be required to discover all of the contributing factors to your fatigue. This book is a thirty-day program to educate you on how to take an active part in trying to solve this mystery. It will also help you discover how to restore your body's capacity for energy and vitality.

There is no "Magic Pill" or "Miracle Cure" for fatigue. There are **multiple** health and lifestyle choices you can make to give you much greater energy and vitality. You have to practice the **majority** of these health habits in order to experience your greatest possible level of improvement. Doctors cannot make these changes for you.

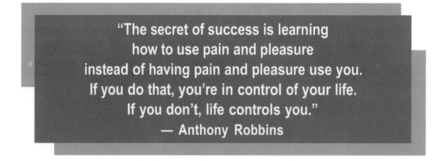

"The secret of success is learning
how to use pain and pleasure
instead of having pain and pleasure use you.
If you do that, you're in control of your life.
If you don't, life controls you."
— Anthony Robbins

For people with serious fatigue problems, restoring the level of energy you desire can certainly take longer than a month. However, by the end of one month the overwhelming majority of my patients and Health-Coaching clients see dramatic changes on multiple levels. This encourages them and lets them know they are making positive steps in the right direction. It is my hope that each person reading this book will adopt these health and lifestyle habits for not just one month, but for their entire life.

One of the basic concepts taught to any physician, is that ninety percent of the diagnosis comes from a patient's history. In my eighteen years of practice, I have taken that concept to heart. I have studied anything I could get my hands on to help me understand what causes symptoms to occur. I became a "medical detective," constantly digging for clues in the patient's history, lab work and symptoms.

I came to recognize that symptoms are not a defect but a message about your health. They serve us best if we seek to understand the message rather than "shooting the messenger" by trying to squelch the symptom.

Imagine you were told you have cancer in four different parts of the body. Treatment will require multiple operations and several doses of chemotherapy. What is your belief about your chances for survival? In October 1996, the person receiving that grim news was elite cyclist, **Lance Armstrong**. Certainly, he was scared out of his mind. But he did not just roll over and give up. He fought hard.

Less than three years later, Lance won the most grueling of bike races, the **Tour de France**. In the year 2000, he won it again! Lance's awesome victories are causing medical books to be rewritten. Not only should doctors stop viewing cancer survivors as weaker, but they should begin to realize how strong the human spirit is in recovering from disease and achieving unbelievable levels of personal strength and endurance.

When a person is that ill, many doctors (and their patients) expect the outcome to be fatal. It is the belief in the power of the disease that fulfills the prophecy. When an elite athlete gets sick, sometimes, extraordinary outcomes occur. Their belief in the strength of their bodies often exceeds their belief in the disease. Champion skater, **Scott Hamilton**, is another wonderful example of a triumphant recovery from cancer and a return to the career he loves.

Before beginning this book, the most important idea I want you to grasp is that ***we are all elite at something.*** Each of us has an extremely important mission to fulfill on this earth. In order to achieve our destiny, we need strong minds and bodies.

I do not believe Lance fought back from what some would consider a death sentence, just for his own glory. His victories are inspiration to the millions of cancer sufferers, to regain the hope to fight, survive and thrive. I guarantee you he gets much greater satisfaction hearing from thousands of cancer survivors than he does receiving a pat on the back from a fellow competitor.

I want you to be healthier and more energetic – not so you can admire yourself in the mirror, but so you can accomplish something remarkable. You have great blessings to share with your loved ones, your community, or perhaps, people on the other side of the world who have difficulties. You will never achieve your highest potential if you are making changes just to benefit yourself. Find a person, place or cause on which to shine your light. Use this book to make your light shine brighter!

> "The capacity for hope is the most significant fact of life. It provides human beings with a sense of destination and the energy to get started."
> — Norman Cousins

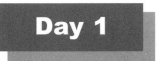

"Most of the important things in the world have been accomplished by people who have kept on trying when there seemed to be no hope at all."

—Dale Carnegie

Are You Tired or Toxic?

When you are tired, depleted, toxic and stressed, hope is the most valuable commodity. Nothing is worse than a doctor who squelches a patient's hope with the statement, ***"There's nothing more that can be done for your condition."*** Please recognize that this statement is ***only*** correct when ***one small word*** is inserted. This sentence should always be stated, "There's nothing more *I* can do for your condition." It is impossible for any single doctor or branch of health care to know everything.

When I made that statement, you probably thought of a patient with a serious disease such as cancer. As a chiropractor, I can not tell you how many patients I have seen who were told by their doctors to "just live with" minor neck pains, headaches or low back pains even though they were relatively easy to correct with chiropractic techniques.

With the vast array of medical therapies and health knowledge available today, each doctor can only study a small piece of the puzzle. My own healing came from multiple sources. Most medical doctors do not have enough experience with alternative medical practices to know the abilities of a chiropractor or naturopath. Many doctors have not learned how to apply nutrition to health problems, just as most chiropractors or acupuncturists do not know what goes on in a surgery or how to dose medications.

We are starting this healing journey with an understanding of toxicity, because this area of health care is often overlooked in our busy world of high-tech machines and "wonder-drugs." So many people are severely fatigued today, because health care professionals pay little attention to helping people improve the body's detoxification efforts. Detoxification was a big medical focus in the early 1900's. In the past one hundred years, our planet has become extremely toxic, yet we have failed to recognize the need to augment our body's incredible self-healing mechanisms.

There is no way to completely grasp what needs to be detoxified by our bodies today compared to our ancestors in the "horse and buggy" days. Yet, at least once a week, I encounter someone who still thinks their body ought to be just fine by eating a "good diet." This chapter will delve into numerous ways our bodies have an increased toxic burden that I believe can no longer be managed with simply diet alone.

An overburden on our organs of detoxification is one of the major causes of fatigue. Helping our cells, organs and tissues adequately rid wastes is the most important factor in raising our energy and vitality--more important than nourishment itself. In order to convert toxic substances into a nontoxic form that can be safely excreted, a number of metabolic reactions must occur. These reactions require a rich supply of vitamins, minerals, antioxidants and phytonutrients.

SOURCES OF TOXIC BURDEN:

- Intestinal dysfunction: constipation, diarrhea (harmful germs, parasites), inadequate digestion, loss of normal intestinal flora
- Food allergies and intolerances
- Overconsumption of congesting foods such as dairy and flour products
- Food additives, colorings, hydrogenated fats
- Impaired function of detoxification organs
- Inadequate consumption of foods rich in chlorophyll and other phytonutrients to neutralize free radicals and cleanse the blood
- Lack of activity and exercise
- Shallow breathing
- Air pollution, cigarette smoke
- Environmental toxins: home cleaning products, home and lawn insecticide exposure
- Chlorine, heavy metals, pesticides, herbicides, etc. in drinking water
- Medications

ORGANS OF DETOXIFICATION

The primary organs of detoxification include the colon, liver, kidneys, lungs and skin. The lungs eliminate toxic gases that accumulate in our bloodstream from normal metabolism or the air we breathe. Lack of exercise and shallow breathing from increased stress contribute greatly to excessive toxicity.

The liver detoxifies everything that enters the body via the lungs, skin and digestive tract. This long list includes foods, caffeine, food additives, drugs, alcohol, pesticides and chemical pollutants. In the U.S., we have over ten thousand food and chemical additives in our food supply. The average American eats about fourteen pounds of additives per year. These include colorings, preservatives, flavorings, emulsifiers, humectants and antimicrobials.

Toxins neutralized by the liver are then eliminated either by the kidneys and bladder if they are water-soluble or through the bile if they are fat-soluble. Bile toxins are then excreted by the feces. The colon eliminates the end-products of digestion. The skin eliminates toxins through sweat and pores.

CONSIDER THE AMOUNT OF ENVIRONMENTAL POISONS RELEASED INTO OUR ENVIRONMENT IN JUST ONE YEAR (1996):

- Over 248 million pounds of industrial chemicals were dumped into public sewage.
- More than 418 million pounds of chemicals were released into the ground, threatening our natural ground water resouces.
- Over forty-five million pounds of chemicals were discharged into surface waters such as lakes and rivers.
- More than one trillion pounds of air emissions were released into the atmosphere.
- The grand total of chemical pollutants released into the U.S. environment, in one year, was enough to fill a line of semi-trailers parked bumper to bumper from Los Angeles to Des Moines, Iowa!

Detoxification is a big job for our bodies. When the organs of elimination are not working properly, the skin often shows abnormalities of color, texture, rashes, itching, cysts or blemishes. Deficiencies in lung function cause the skin to appear pale or ashen. Liver problems make the skin yellow or amber and may cause itching. Kidney dysfunction can cause dark circles or swelling of the lower eyelid.

Colon dysfunction often results in blemishes, rashes or eczema. Inadequate digestion or an abnormal bacterial flora in the colon can result in a diaper rash in infants or an itchy rectum in adults. An excess of hard-to-digest fats, such as hydrogenated fats, can cause little fatty cysts known as lipomas, which frequently appear on the back. An excess of mucus in the nose, sinuses, throat, and/or lungs often comes from poor digestion or an excess of mucus-causing foods such as dairy and flour products.

Conquer Fatigue in 30 Days will teach you many ways to minimize toxicity and maximize the body's methods of detoxification. One of the ways I measure the seriousness of a clients' initial problems and their subsequent progress is with the following Toxicity Questionnaire. This questionnaire rates the frequency and severity of symptoms with numbers. It has been used by hundreds of "Functional Medicine" practitioners as a "before" and "after" assessment. You will take this test again in ***Day 30 - Graduation Day***.

This questionnaire is a starting place to discover the various areas of your body overburdened by toxicity. A total point score over twenty-five points indicates you need some improvement in detoxification. Very often, when people start to feel better, they forget how bad they once felt. You will be surprised at the end of the program how many symptoms have been improved or resolved.

"Concerning all acts of initiative and creation, there is one elementary truth – that the moment one definitely commits oneself, then Providence moves, too."
— Werner von Braun

TOXICITY QUESTIONNAIRE

©1997 HealthComm International, Inc. and Immuno Laboratories, Inc. Permission to reprint R9/12/97

Rate the following symptoms based upon your health profile for the past thirty days

Point scale

0 – *Never* or *almost never* have the symptom
1 - *Occasionally* have it, effect is *not severe*
2 - *Occasionally* have it, effect is *severe*
3 - *Frequently* have it, effect is *not severe*
4 - *Frequently* have it, effect is *severe*

HEAD
_____ Headaches
_____ Faintness
_____ Dizziness
_____ Insomnia   Total _____

EYES
_____ Watery or itchy eyes
_____ Swollen, reddened, or sticky eyelids
_____ Bags or dark circles under eyes
_____ Blurred or tunnel vision (does not include near– or far-sightedness)
                                                                        Total _____

EARS
_____ Itchy ears
_____ Earaches, ear infections
_____ Drainage from ear
_____ Ringing in ears, hearing loss   Total _____

NOSE
_____ Stuffy nose
_____ Sinus problems
_____ Hay fever
_____ Sneezing attacks
_____ Excessive mucus formation   Total _____

MOUTH /THROAT
_____ Chronic coughing
_____ Gagging, frequent need to clear throat
_____ Sore throat, hoarseness, loss of voice
_____ Swollen or discolored tongue, gums, lips
_____ Canker sores   Total _____

SKIN
_____ Acne
_____ Hives, rashes, dry skin
_____ Hair loss
_____ Flushing, hot flashes
_____ Excessive sweating   Total _____

HEART
_____ Irregular or skipped heartbeat
_____ Rapid or pounding heartbeat
_____ Chest pain   Total _____

LUNGS
- _____ Chest congestion
- _____ Asthma, bronchitis
- _____ Shortness of breath
- _____ Difficulty breathing   Total _____

DIGESTIVE TRACT
- _____ Nausea, vomiting
- _____ Diarrhea
- _____ Constipation
- _____ Bloated feeling
- _____ Belching, passing gas
- _____ Heartburn
- _____ Intestinal/stomach pain   Total _____

JOINTS/ MUSCLE
- _____ Pain or aches in joints
- _____ Arthritis
- _____ Stiffness or limitation of movement
- _____ Pain or aches in muscles
- _____ Feeling of weakness or tiredness   Total _____

WEIGHT
- _____ Binge eating/drinking
- _____ Craving certain foods
- _____ Excessive weight
- _____ Compulsive eating
- _____ Water retention
- _____ Underweight   Total _____

ENERGY/ ACTIVITY
- _____ Fatigue, sluggishness
- _____ Apathy, lethargy
- _____ Hyperactivity
- _____ Restlessness   Total _____

MIND
- _____ Poor memory
- _____ Confusion, poor comprehension
- _____ Poor concentration
- _____ Poor physical coordination
- _____ Difficulty in making decisions
- _____ Stuttering or stammering
- _____ Slurred speech
- _____ Learning disabilities   Total _____

EMOTIONS
- _____ Mood swings
- _____ Anxiety, fear, nervousness
- _____ Anger, irritability, aggressiveness
- _____ Depression   Total _____

OTHER
- _____ Frequent illness
- _____ Frequent or urgent urination
- _____ Genital itch or discharge   Total _____

GRAND TOTAL _____

The following are examples from a few clients who achieved a high degree of symptom reversal:

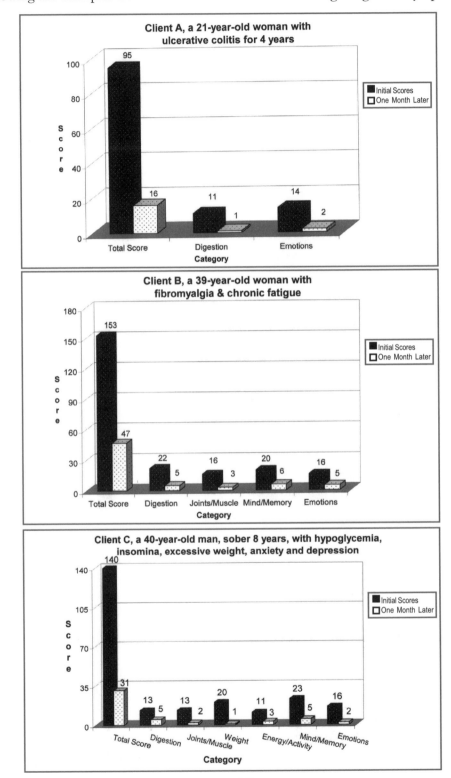

TODAY'S ACTIVITY

First, take a moment to list your five most significant health problems, ranking the most troublesome first. Some examples might be fatigue, constipation, arthritis, depression, etc. You will have a chance to write down some of your other symptoms in subsequent chapters. Consider what you believe to be the cause of these problems.

<u>Symptoms</u>   <u>Causes</u>

1. _____

2. _____

3. _____

4. _____

5. _____

Now, let's shift the focus from *"symptoms you don't want"* to *"how you would like to feel."* Take a moment to visualize what you wish to happen in the future regarding your health:

What are your health goals over the next thirty days?

_____

_____

_____

What are your health goals in three months?

_____

_____

_____

If you believed there were no limits on your health, what would be your health goals in one year?

_____

_____

_____

I sincerely hope you set some far-reaching goals and can start to believe that you do not have to live a life of fatigue and low vitality. You are ready to embark on the most important journey of your life. Taking charge of your nutrition, lifestyle and stress is the only "insurance" that brings you true health.

> "I've learned that to ignore the facts
> does not change the facts."
> — Andy Rooney

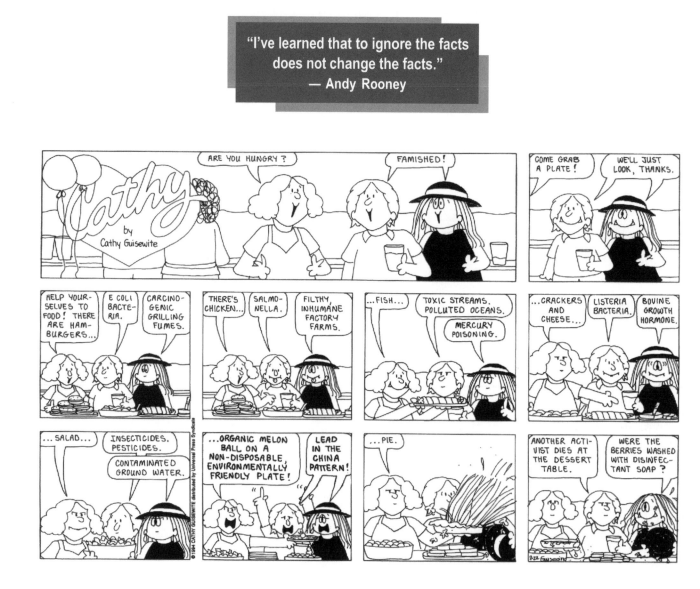

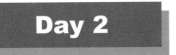

Day 2

"It's easier to prepare and prevent,
than to repair and repent."
— Unknown

The Big 3--
Multivitamins, Antioxidants, Essential Fats

Helping people recover from years of nutrient depletion is a very complex problem that involves a multitude of factors. Many of these factors involve food and beverage choices. A tired or exhasted person develops various eating habits, which involve choosing things that are fast and easy, but not necessarily the most nutritious.

It is overwhelming for many fatigued individuals to consider changes in the way they select and prepare foods. I have had many people tell me at the beginning of their program that they do not cook and absolutely will not cook. This is why I have introduced dietary changes in this book gradually and in a specific order. The first place I start is having people begin a high-quality nutritional supplementation program that "covers the bases." This allows people to begin feeling and thinking better, so they can arrive at a place where they are more willing to improve the quality of their meals.

The following list includes some of many factors associated with fatigue that are related to the depletion of nutrients:

FACTORS RELATED TO DEPLETION AND THE INABILITY TO PRODUCE ENERGY

- Anemia, due to malnutrition, pregnancy, disease or blood loss
- Depletion of nutrients from agricultural soils
- Inadequate consumption of fresh fruits and vegetables
- The avoidance of all fats, including the essential fats
- Inadequate protein consumption
- Overconsumption of nutrient-robbing foods such as sugar, white flour, caffeine, alcohol and soda pop
- Poor digestive function and inadequate absorption of nutrients
- Low thyroid function (hypothyroidism)
- Hypoglycemia, dysglycemia and hyperglycemia (diabetes)
- Infection or impaired immune function
- Medications that deplete nutrients
- Serious degenerative diseases such as cancer and autoimmune disorders

The three supplements I consider most important are a high quality multivitamin/mineral, a broad-spectrum antioxidant formula and essential fatty acids, most frequently the omega-3 variety. Supplementing with the "Big 3" often eliminates about eighty percent of most peoples' symptoms. Later, we can focus on certain individual nutrients that some may need more than the average person.

The mission statement of my clinic is *"To ethically teach and inspire people to choose health strategies that promote wellness, vitality and longevity and minimize the need for drugs and surgery."* Minimizing the need for drugs also relates to how I feel about nutritional supplements. My goal is to help people use the fewest products possible. Sometimes people take a wide assortment of nutritional products they have read articles about, and later forget why they bought them. It is not unusual to find people taking a dozen or more products.

Sometimes, people may be doing more harm than good by taking products that throw off their vitamin and mineral balances. One of the most common mistakes is to take just one or two minerals without taking a multivitamin. Most commonly it is calcium or zinc. Whenever you take an individual mineral alone it impacts every other mineral in your body, causing each level to go up or down.

For example, with calcium being added to orange juice or other foods it is common for people to be ingesting too much calcium in respect to other minerals. Excessive calcium can cause a magnesium deficiency and aggravate conditions such as high blood pressure, asthma, and constipation. Taking a multivitamin/mineral can often eliminate the need for extra calcium or prevent it from creating imbalance when it is taken along with the multivitamin/mineral.

Another common vitamin fad is B-complex formulas, which contain every B vitamin at twenty-five, fifty, seventy-five, or one hundred milligrams. This was a bizarre marketing gimmick that started over thirty years ago and continues today. A well-researched multivitamin or B- complex formula has very different levels of each B vitamin, as you would find in nature. These differences are pivotal in providing balance for the desired effect. An imbalanced formula may cause problems with brain and heart function.

RECOMMENDED DAILY ALLOWANCES

If the majority of Americans were to compare their diets against the meager **Recommended Daily Allowance (RDA)** guidelines for vitamins and minerals they would fall very short. According to the **U.S. Department of Agriculture (USDA)**, more than eighty percent of women and more than seventy percent of men eat less than two-thirds of the **RDA** for one or more nutrients. The **Standard American Diet**, aptly nicknamed **SAD**, is rich in fried foods, hydrogenated fats and nutrient-depleting junk foods.

Keep in mind the **RDA** guidelines were developed in the 1940's, and rarely get revised. The **Food and Nutrition Board** of the **National Academy of Sciences** reviews the **RDA's** every ten years, but the **FDA** has the final word on revisions. Unfortunately, changes in the **RDA's** are difficult because of political, scientific, and economic issues. It is difficult to get a consensus from scientists. Economically, it is even more difficult for the United States to raise the bar for malnutrition because so many more people would then qualify for government aid.

The **RDA's** are the bare minimum you need to prevent ***known nutritional deficiency diseases***. They have nothing to do with ***optimal*** levels or amounts that prevent the earlier, first symptoms of disease. They do not take into account that some people can have an extraordinary need for individual nutrients based on genetic differences, state of health, taking drugs or exposure to toxins.

Babies are never born with more minerals than their parents. The shortage of a mineral such as chromium, can be part of the reason why a disease like diabetes has such strong "genetic" tendencies. Some doctors now believe that nutritional intervention can delay or prevent such genetic expression.

The following chart has a short list of the more commonly used products that cause nutrient depletion.

NUTRIENT – DEPLETING SUBSTANCES	
Reprinted by permission from *Healthy Answers*, Winter 2000, **Advanced Nutrition Publications**	
Product:	**What it Depletes From Your Body:**
Alcohol (includes drugs containing alcohol, such as cough syrups)	Vitamins A, B_1, B_2, biotin, choline, niacin, folic acid, magnesium
Antacids (containing aluminum & calcium)	Iron, phosphorus, thiamin
Anticoagulants (e.g., coumadin)	Vitamins A, K
Antiepileptic drugs and sedatives	Calcium, folic acid, vitamins D, K
Antihistamines	Vitamin C
Aspirin	Vitamin C
Barbituates	Vitamins A, C, D, folic acid
Birth control pills & estrogen replacement	Folic acid, vitamin B_6
Caffeine	Vitamin B_1, inositol, biotin, calcium, iron, potassium, zinc
Cholesterol-lowering drugs	Vitamins A, D, E, K
Cimetidine	Vitamin B_1
Diuretics (non-potassium sparing)	Potassium, magnesium, B complex
Nicotine	Vitamins C, B_1, folic acid, calcium
Penicillin (any form)	Vitamins B_6, niacin, K
Soda pop	Vitamins B_1, B_2, B_3, B_5, B_6, lipoic acid, manganese, biotin, iron, magnesium, sulfur, Coenzyme Q-10, calcium
Steroids	Vitamins B_6, C, D
Sugar	Vitamins B_1, B_2, B_3, B_5, B_6, lipoic acid, manganese, biotin, iron, magnesium, sulfur, Coenzyme Q-10
Tetracyclines	Vitamin K, calcium, magnesium, iron

DISEASE PREVENTION

Only about ten percent of people heed the advice of the **National Cancer Institute** to eat five or more fruits and vegetables per day. Even our school lunch program has expanded the definition of vegetable by including ketchup as a vegetable serving to meet dietary standards.

Four of the top ten causes of health-related deaths in the U.S. – cancer, heart disease, stroke, and diabetes – are related to diet. A study of 42,000 women, published in the April 26, 2000 *Journal of the American Medical Association*, showed that eating a wide variety of healthy foods can result in a thirty percent decrease in risk of dying from cancer, heart disease and stroke. The study looked at the frequency of consumption of twenty-three recommended foods in the categories of fruits, vegetables, whole grains and low-fat meat and dairy products.

The power of nutritional supplementation was also made very apparent in a recent fifteen-year study on nearly ninety thousand female nurses, reported in the October, 1997 issue of the *Annals of Internal Medicine*. There was an astounding *seventy-five percent less incidence of colon cancer* in those who were taking a multivitamin/mineral for the entire fifteen years.

The consequences of SAD are glaringly apparent. Obesity rates have exploded in this country in the past twenty years, now affecting thirty-three percent of adults. Children are also faring poorly with about twenty-five percent of children being overweight or at risk for being overweight. The percentage of children who are overweight has doubled since 1980. A **World Health Organization** study of more than 120,000 children in twenty-eight countries found that American kids exercise less often and eat more junk food than kids in most other places. Two-thirds of youngsters in the U.S. exercise less than two hours per week. A staggering thirty-one percent of them reported eating french fries *every day*!

The bottom line is: The majority of Americans need to improve their eating habits and cover their bases with nutrient supplementation. Doctors need to start encouraging their patients to use multivitamins, especially women who are sexually active and liable to become pregnant. In the past fifty years, many doctors made their patients feel like taking vitamins was a foolish waste of money. They insisted that we received all the necessary nutrients in plentiful amounts in a "well-balanced" diet. Of those individuals who truly understand what a well-balanced diet is, few actually choose the correct foods on a regular basis.

Another factor, affecting nutrient content in foods, is the problem of mineral-depleted soils in the U.S. for at least the past sixty years. Most fruits and vegetables will contain vitamins no matter how poorly they are grown. Vitamins are manufactured by the plants. Minerals, however, will only be in the plants if they are found in the soil. Therefore, since modern agriculture utilizes primarily nitrogen, phosphorus and potassium (NPK) with calcium fertilizers, crops are drawing every last mineral out of the soils. NPK offers nothing to ensure the plants will have adequate amounts of zinc, iron, manganese, chromium, vanadium, selenium, etc.

Organic farming practices are known as sustainable agriculture because they nourish the soils with decomposed organic matter in order to provide minerals and other nutrients that make the plants healthier and more resistant to disease. This allows an organic farmer to avoid pesticides and commercial fertilizers. This is comparable to what happens in humans. Those who are well nourished and have adequate mineral stores will fend off infections and disease much more effectively.

Organic farming practices also encourage a healthier microorganism balance in the soil. These are important for the fixation of minerals into plants. Commercial farming chemicals kill off the soil's healthy microorganisms and worms, thus creating ecological imbalances.

When people grew up closer to the land they wasted nothing and consumed the organs from animals. American Indians would immediately eat the adrenal gland from the buffalo they killed. Livers, hearts, brains, kidneys and even intestines have been consumed. These mineral-rich organs were our grandparents' "multivitamins." Americans now consume only the muscle from animals. The livers stopped being consumed because of toxicity issues from all the drugs given to livestock. The other organs are just considered unpalatable to today's picky eaters.

Today, most Americans are only willing to consume their organ and glandular tissues in pill form. I use products with my patients that contain tissues from lungs, kidneys, heart, liver, adrenals, thyroid, etc. **Metagenics** uses only organ and glandular products from New Zealand to avoid toxicity problems.

MULTIVITAMINS

When choosing any supplement, quality is the most important factor to consider. You have to choose a brand that uses high quality raw materials, proper ratios and balance of nutrients, as well as capsules or tableting agents that are non-toxic and not irritating to the gastrointestinal tract. Choosing a product with the lowest price will often sacrifice quality in many of those areas.

Trying to decide which brand is best when you have no knowledge who owns the company and how much care and concern they put into the quality of their products makes your choice very difficult.

Do not rely on advertising to steer you in the right direction. Many companies spend plenty of money creating the public perception that they are the latest and greatest. My general rule of advice is - the more a company spends on advertising, the less they spend on the actual product.

Many people have the impression that nutritional products sold in health food stores are better than those sold in drug stores. Many of the vitamin brands sold in health food stores have been bought, in the last decade, by the same drug companies whose products are sold in pharmacies. Very few independent brands remain.

I use three different nutrition companies in my practice, all of which primarily sell to licensed physicians and are independent brands. The company I use most, **Metagenics**, is the most popular brand among doctors who utilize nutrition in North America. More doctors choose **Metagenics** because we are able to trust that their products have solid nutritional research, quality, purity and safety behind them. **Metagenics** also has two product lines sold in health food stores under the names "**Ethical Nutrients**" and "**Unipro.**" The **Unipro** line specializes in supplements for athletes.

WHY AREN'T YOU TAKING A MULTIVITAMIN/MINERAL?

Many people have avoided taking multivitamins for a variety of reasons. We have already mentioned the discouragement of doctors and the mistaken belief that our diets have everything we need. Some people have tried products that gave them an upset stomach. Others have heard reports that taking all the minerals at the same time causes a competition for absorption. Still others have noticed an increase in appetite or weight gain when taking some multivitamins.

These are valid complaints with some products on the market. In general, I teach patients that the multivitamins with a one-per-day dosage are usually less expensive, inorganic minerals that can be irritating to the stomach and poorly absorbed. Cheap ingredients allow for a lower retail price and mislead the consumer into thinking they are getting a "good deal." In reality, there is nothing more expensive than a supplement you cannot absorb.

Inorganic minerals often compete with each other for absorption. The type of minerals found in Metagenics nutritional products are a special amino acid chelate, patented by **Albion Laboratories** of Utah. Each mineral is bound to an amino acid protein to improve its absorption and to prevent the competitive absorption found with free, inorganic minerals.

The only disadvantage is it disappoints people who have been conditioned to believe they can get everything they need in a one-per-day dosage. Binding each mineral to an amino acid makes it a much bigger molecule and drives the daily dosage up to around six per day. **Metagenics** sells their multivitamin in both capsule and tablet form. They also make a powdered form for people who dislike taking pills or have difficulty swallowing. Many of my patients who had experienced increased appetite or weight gain with previous products do not have that problem with **Metagenics** brand.

VITAMIN FRAUD

Another unfortunate reality to the vitamin business is the dishonesty and sometimes, outright fraud in which some companies engage. Some formulas do not contain the listed potency and others do not contain even a single ounce of the primary ingredients.

Since the **Dietary Supplements Health and Education Act** of 1994, the **Food and Drug Administration** has less ability to regulate the supplement industry the way it regulates prescription and over-the-counter drugs. The **FDA** does not have the resources to check every product on the market for labeling, potency, quality, freedom from contaminants or the ability to absorb the product. Some of the products do not dissolve and are visible on abdominal x-rays.

Vitamin companies are only required to follow the "good manufacturing practices" (GMP's) of the food industry. More reputable companies, such as **Metagenics**, adhere to many of the more stringent GMP's of the pharmaceutical industry.

About ten years ago, **Metagenics** found a multivitamin with similar ingredients to theirs for a retail price of about $9. Their product at the time was around $25. They did a cost analysis of everything listed on Brand X's label and found the raw materials cost over $14. Since no company could afford to sell its product for $5 less than it costs to make it, Brand X was obviously lying about what was in their product.

In 1990, the ***Journal of Obstetrics and Gynecology*** printed an analysis of eleven different brands of acidophilus products. Five of the brands listed as many as three additional species of bacteria in their products.

Tests showed:
- All contained only a single species of bacteria.
- Nine of the eleven had a bacteria that looks and tastes like acidophilus known as *Lactobacillus casei*, which is most commonly used to make cheese.
- Only two products contained acidophilus, but one falsely claimed to have contained two species of bacteria and the other claimed three species.

Therefore, all eleven brands did not meet their label claim and ***nine contained no acidophilus***. Whether this was intentional fraud or just not having their raw materials properly verified is unknown.

Similar studies, done on St. John's Wort, have shown everything from excessive to inadequate ingredients and in some cases, the absence of any detectable St. John's Wort herb. My point is, the vitamin industry is huge and vastly unregulated. Some companies use this lack of regulation to their advantage and accrue enormous profits to the misfortune of the trusting consumer. Remember the old saying, "If it sounds too good to be true, it probably is."

According to **TIME Magazine**, July 31, 2000, there is now an independent laboratory in White Plains, N.Y., that is trying to position itself as the "Consumer Reports of the supplement industry." Their web site, **www.consumerlab.com,** lists some brands that have passed their criteria for potency, purity, bioavailability and consistency.

TODAY'S ACTIVITY

The following is a list of criteria you should consider when choosing a multivitamin-mineral. Check this list against your present multivitamin.

Does Your Multiple Vitamin/Mineral Supplement Pass The Test?

1. Include balanced antioxidants?

A balance of various antioxidants is critical in order to achieve the beneficial effects attributed to them such as protection from free radical damage, anti-aging, improved immune function, improved cardiovascular health, etc. while receiving the documented benefits of their synergistic actions. Balanced antioxidants include:

Mixed Carotenoids   Yes   No

Natural beta-carotene, balanced within a broad spectrum of carotenoids, is preferred over synthetic. Beta-carotene is only one of over fifty naturally occurring carotenoids (like lutein, zeaxanthin, alpha-carotene, etc.) found in food. Large doses of a single carotenoid may inhibit the utilization of others, thus inhibiting their effects. Beta-carotene alone has been implicated as a tumor promoter in the lungs of smokers in two controversial studies. A product listing of "beta-carotene" means that it is likely synthetic beta-carotene alone unless it is identified as "mixed carotenoids." Foods high in natural carotenoids (also called phytonutrients) are thought to protect against cancer and heart disease, as well as other diseases.

Vitamin C   Yes   No

Ascorbic acid (vitamin C) is a critical antioxidant for human health. In addition, it potentiates and preserves the effectiveness of other antioxidants.

Natural Vitamin E   Yes   No

The chemical names for natural vitamin E are d-Alpha tocopherol or d-Alpha tocopheryl acetate. Studies show that natural vitamin E is more effective than the synthetic version (dl-alpha tocopherol).

Bioflavonoid Complex   Yes   No

Hundreds of different bioflavonoids are found in fruits and vegetables – giving them their bright colors. They provide powerful antioxidant protection, as well as serving other important preventative health roles.

Quercetin   Yes   No

Quercetin not only helps prevent the oxidation of beta-carotene, it is one of the most powerful and most researched of the bioflavonoids. Increased levels of oxidized beta-carotene in the lungs is thought to be the reason that synthetic beta-carotene may promote tumor growth in the lungs of smokers.

Selenium   Yes   No

Selenium is essential to the production of glutathione peroxidase, an important antioxidant enzyme produced within the body. In addition, selenium supplementation has been linked to reduced rates of colorectal, lung and prostate cancers.

Superoxide Dismutase (SOD) Pecursor Blend   Yes   No

SOD is an important antioxidant enzyme necessary for combating potent free radicals in the body. Supplements of SOD are thought to be less effective than simply supplying its precursors. By providing true amino acid chelate precursors (zinc, copper and manganese) SOD activity can be increased.

TODAY'S ACTIVITY CONTINUED

2. Include true mineral amino acid chelates?   Yes   No

Some mineral salts such as sulfates, carbonates, citrates, gluconates, fumerates, lactates, etc. may have limited absorption or negatively affect the absorption of other minerals. They are more suscep- tible to absorption interference from the diet, and may be the cause of stomach and/or intestinal discomfort. If the minerals in a supplement are not true amino acid chelates, they are likely non- chelated mineral salts. True mineral amino acid chelates (e.g., glycinate, histindinate, lysinate, etc.) do not create the same inhibition of absorption that is seen in inorganic minerals, and are not as affected by dietary factors that interfere with absorption. True amino acid chelates are usually patented Albion® chelates, since Albion® holds most of the patents for amino acid chelates. The label should reference the Albion® name or patent numbers to be sure they are true chelates.

3. Include a full range of ratio-balanced B vitamins?   Yes   No

B vitamins are interdependent, and a deficiency of one can often mean others will be low. A multiple should contain the full complex (B_1, B_2, pantothenic acid, biotin, folic acid, niacin, B_6, and B_{12}). In addition, a ratio balance of these should be evident rather than an arbitrary consistent level like twenty- five or fifty milligrams each.

4. Avoid toxicity risk?   Yes   No

Because a multi is something that one takes everyday, rather than for short periods of time, it is important that nutrients with toxicity risk are kept at a safe level for long-term daily consumption.
   a. manganese (1 mg daily)
   b. chromium (200 mcg daily)
   c. vitamin A (5000 IU daily)
   d. selenium (200 mcg daily)

5. Avoid ingredients with gastric irritation risk?   Yes   No

Certain substances commonly used in dietary supplements can irritate the stomach and/or intes- tines. This may not only cause discomfort, but may also reduce the absorption of both supplemental and dietary nutrients.
   a. no iron, zinc or magnesium as sulfates or carbonates
   b. no calcium carbonate
   c. no synthetic excipients (e.g., talc, polyvinyl perilodone, etc.)

6. Avoid ingredients with allergic/hypersensitivity risk?   Yes   No

Allergic or hypersensitivity reactions may account for adverse reactions to dietary supplements. A high quality product will take measures to avoid common allergens.
   a. no artificial colors, flavors, sweeteners or preservatives
   b. no yeast, soy, wheat, milk, eggs, sugar, lactose, or salt

If you checked "yes" to every question, your multi has passed the test--
it is of high quality and safe to take.

PRENATAL VITAMINS

Another important topic with respect to multivitamins, is prenatal vitamins. Please do not skip this section just because you have no plans to have children. Adequate prenatal nutrition affects all of us in regard to insurance costs for both mother and baby and the need to provide special education for children with birth defects. Please pass this information on to a pregnant woman who needs to make informed choices.

In America, prenatals are typically the only nutritional product covered by insurance. They are important from a public health standpoint, since it is very costly to care for a child who develops birth defects from a malnourished pregnancy.

Unfortunately, many of the prescription brands are woefully inadequate, deficient primarily in both major minerals and trace minerals. Apparently there is no formula standard for minerals in prenatals by the pharmaceutical industry. Most contain no more than four or five of the eleven minerals that are important for a healthy mother and baby. Some contain as little as *one* mineral.

CASE STUDY

This was the case with one of our new patients who came in for back problems just as she was about to undergo her second attempt at in vitro fertilization (IVF). From my perspective, if she is having difficulty conceiving and even more difficulty having success with an expensive procedure like IVF, the quality of her nourishment needs to be a primary consideration.

Her prenatal vitamin contained just one mineral – iron (see prenatal comparison chart, page twenty-one). It contained no calcium, magnesium, zinc, iodine, chromium, manganese, etc. She was not pleased when we compared her "prescription" formula to our "over the counter" **Metagenics** prenatal formula (**Fem PreNatal®**). She immediately changed her prenatals and luckily, this time her IVF was successful.

If pregnancy is the most nutritionally demanding time in a woman's life, why are most prenatals severely deficient in ingredients commonly found in the average multivitamin available on the market? Most prenatals also contain inorganic minerals that irritate the stomach. Since many pregnant women have trouble keeping anything down, it makes no sense to use a product that may further irritate the stomach.

What are the consequences of malnourishing our mothers and future generations? Over the years, I have had scores of women tell me that they have never felt healthy since a pregnancy several years prior. How many of the "normal side effects" of pregnancy such as premature contractions, gestational diabetes, toxemia and postpartum depression are related to poor nutritional support? In 1999, singer **Marie Osmond** suffered a very public bout of postpartum depression. Some researchers estimate that this condition affects as many as eighty percent of new mothers.

How many problems with babies such as low birth weights, prematurity, birth defects, frequent illnesses and ADD are caused by this inadequate nourishment? When you ask an obstetrician or pharmacist about prenatal vitamins, their focus is on the level of folic acid, calcium and iron. Every other ingredient in a multivitamin or prenatal is considered superfluous.

An article on birth defects in **USA Today** on April 12, 2000, stated that birth defects are still the leading cause of infant death in the USA and are also a major cause of disability in young people. **Jennifer Howse**, president of the **March of Dimes** was quoted as saying, "This problem of birth defects is not going away. We don't know what causes about eighty percent of the birth defects."

The article also discussed that only eight states have competent tracking programs to study birth defects. Seventeen states have no tracking programs for birth defects. **Dr. Lynn Goldman**, a pediatrician and lead researcher in this study states, "We have no information on the developmental effects of more than seventy-eight percent of the 2,863 high-production-volume chemicals produced in the U.S. We do know that of the top one hundred chemicals that are released into our environment, forty-two are suspected and recognized as affecting prenatal development."

California is one of the few states to investigate autism rates. A survey by its **Department of Developmental Services** found a 210 percent rise in the number of autistic children enrolled in state programs between 1987 and 1998. A researcher called it an *"autism epidemic."*

Despite the evidence that we need to be more proactive about enhancing the health of both mothers and their babies, on the web site for a major U.S. health instituation, an obstetrician offers the following response to the question, ***"What about nutritional supplements (during pregnancy)?"*** Response: ***"A healthy, well-balanced diet will usually supply the extra nutrients needed during pregnancy. There is one big exception, however. We definitely recommend that a woman take folate or folic acid (one of the B vitamins) in the months before she becomes pregnant and in the early stages of pregnancy."***

Inadequate training in nutrition of our nation's medical doctors has been typical for many decades. In 1995, only twenty-five of the nation's 125 medical schools had even a single course in nutrition. The United States was the last of the major industrialized nations to recognize that all women of childbearing age should be taking folic acid. How can our doctors possibly understand the significance of sub-optimal levels of nutrients if they have never been taught the biochemical consequences of these deficiencies?

Unfortunately, pregnant women assume their doctors are aware of every aspect of their prenatal health care. They expect their prenatal vitamin, being prescribed by their doctor and paid for by insurance, to be the highest standard of medical care.

What is the role of the pharmaceutical industry in prenatal formulations? Surely the doctors are trusting drug companies to put together a product that provides the best possible nutrition for pregnant women. Drug companies employ some of the best biochemists in the world. They have far more knowledge about nutrition than any doctor. Perhaps prenatals have been considered a low priority and have not received much attention during the explosive growth of nutrition knowledge over the last fifty years.

Maybe drug companies are limited by the constraints of insurance companies who are being "penny-wise and pound-foolish." The products with few ingredients are undoubtedly cheaper. But are the health consequences of ***not*** providing these important nutrients costing them billions of dollars? Many of these ingredients have established RDA's for pregnancy so why are they not ***mandatory*** in prenatals?

This is the problem when business people instead of scientists and doctors make policy issues about what they will pay for in something as crucial to our public health as prenatal vitamins. A progressive insurance company needs to lead the way in paying only for prenatals that have a broad spectrum of nutritional support. It is a very simple change in policy that could have a ***profound*** effect on the health of mothers and babies.

Nutrition researchers now know at least one third of all enzymes in the body require mineral cofactors for their function. The more active researchers in this field have suggested at least sixty percent of the three thousand known protein enzymes in the human body require minerals for proper function. Lacking these minerals is key to understanding how organ dysfunctions begin to occur, eventually creating symptoms and disease.

Dr. Lucille Hurley and her co-workers at the **University of California at Davis** researched the impact of prenatal nutrition on offspring. This study was published in the **American Journal of Clinical Nutrition** 1982; 35. They placed pregnant mice on a moderately zinc-deficient diet and observed for changes in immune function. The first-generation offspring showed depressed immune function as a result of the mothers' low-zinc diet. Surprisingly, the next two generations of mice also experienced lowered immune function despite the fact that they and the parents were fed a diet containing normal levels of zinc.

It appears the nutritional status of the father can also have genetic implications. According to research published in 1991 by **Dr. Bruce Ames** at the **University of California at Berkeley**, low levels of vitamin C (ten to twenty milligrams per day) can lead to genetic damage in sperm. It is believed such damage to DNA could potentially lead to genetic disorders, birth defects, immune deficiency or cancer in children.

HOW DOES YOUR PRENATAL COMPARE?

We researched some of the more commonly prescribed prenatals. The following table shows the contents of two popular presecription brands compared to **Metagenics Fem Prenatal®**. This product is available without prescription in a form that is gentle on a sensitive stomach. They are conveniently packaged for purse transport when morning sickness forces a pregnant woman to skip breakfast. Dosage is two packets per day of three tablets per packet, taken with meals.

COMPARISON OF PRENATAL VITAMINS			
INGREDIENT	Rx A	FEM PRENATAL®	Rx B
Vitamin A	1000 IU	4,000 IU	Absent
Beta-Carotene	Absent	4,000 IU(mixed carotenoids)	4000 IU
Vitamin D₃	400 IU	400 IU	400 IU
Vitamin E	11 IU	30 IU	30 IU
Folic acid	1 mg	800 mcg	1 mg
B1 (thiamin)	2 mg	3.4 mg	3 mg
B2 (riboflavin)	3 mg	3.4 mg	3 mg
B3 (niacinamide)	20 mg	40 mg (plus Ascorbate)	20 mg
B5 (pantothenic acid)	Absent	20 mg	Absent
B6	10 mg	10 mg	3 mg
B12	12 mcg	12 mcg	8 mcg
Biotin	Absent	300 mcg	Absent
Vitamin C	120 mg	240 mg	120 mg
Vitamin K	Absent	65 mcg	Absent
Calcium	Absent	520 mg	200 mg
Magnesium	Absent	250 mg	Absent
Phosphorus	Absent	160 mg	Absent
Iodine	Absent	175 mcg	150 mcg
Zinc	Absent	25 mg (glycinate)	15 mg (oxide)
Iron	60 mg	30 mg (glycinate)	50 mg (carbonyl)
Copper	Absent	2 mg	Absent
Manganese	Absent	1.2 mg	Absent
Selenium	Absent	12.5 mcg	Absent
Molybdenum	Absent	25 mcg	Absent
Chromium	Absent	25 mcg	Absent
Inositol	Absent	50 mg	Absent
Quercetin	Absent	6 mg	Absent

It is important to discuss some of the benefits of these missing ingredients and how their absence could impact a pregnancy or fetus. Please note that most of these ingredients have established RDA levels for adult women. When I could find a specific RDA for pregnancy I listed it as RDA-P. Again, the RDA is not an optimal level but a bare minimum daily requirement to prevent disease.

I also want to add that **Metagenics** extensively researched the ingredients of their prenatal to be sure they only included those things proven to be safe for pregnancy. Just because an ingredient has never been shown to be harmful, does not prove it is safe, thus products with questionable safety have not been included.

- **Beta-Carotene (as mixed carotenoids)** – Important antioxidant and immune stimulator.
- **B5 (pantothenic acid)** – An important B vitamin that nourishes the adrenal gland - our stress organ. Deficiency can cause adrenal atrophy, fatigue, eczema, depression, headaches, insomnia, nausea, nervousness and hair loss.
- **Biotin (RDA 100 – 200 mcg.)** – A B vitamin that is important in nourishing hair, skin and nails and prevents yeast from turning into its more harmful fungal form. Deficiency can cause dermatitis, depression, fatigue, anemia, hyper-glycemia (diabetes) and hair loss.
- **Vitamin K (RDA 65 mcg.)** – An important vitamin for proper blood clotting. Excessive bleeding can be a complication of labor and could result in needing an emergency hysterectomy following birth.
- **Magnesium (RDA-P – 450 mg)** – One of the most important major minerals in the body, participating in over three hundred metabolic reactions. Deficiency can contribute to chronic musculoskeletal problems, spasm of both smooth (uterus) and skeletal muscles, asthma, hypertension, tachycardia (fast heart rate), PMS, anxiety, confusion, depression, hyperactivity, seizures, constipation, chronic fatigue, etc. More than one percent of pregnant women develop premature uterine contractions and go into labor before thirty-four weeks. Half of those deliver prematurely before thirty-seven weeks. Two 1996 surveys of obstetricians found that about ninety percent treated such patients with weekly steroid injections. Research studies indicate that this treatment might contribute to low birth weight and other unknown risks.
- **Phosphorus (RDA-P – 1200 mg.)** – An important mineral for bone strength. Deficiency can cause loss of appetite, weakness and joint stiffness.
- **Iodine (RDA-P – 125 mcg.)** – Iodine is the primary mineral needed to produce thyroid hormones, and selenium is necessary to convert T4 to T3. Iodine deficiency can cause infertility, miscarriages, premature deliveries and stillbirths. Other hypothyroid symptoms include edema, weight gain, depression, cold hands and feet, low sex drive, fatigue (especially in the mornings), hair and skin changes. Deficiency in infants can cause mental retardation, growth retardation and even death.
- **Zinc (RDA-P– 20 mg.)** – Deficiency causes skin changes, hair loss, recurrent infections and diarrhea. Zinc insuffciencies can also cause insomnia, slow wound healing, dandruff, decreased appetite, and inflammatory bowel disease.
- **Copper** – Used in many enzyme functions involving vitamin C, antioxidants and neurotransmitters. Provides elasticity to blood vessels and skin. Deficiencies include stretch marks, varicose veins, hair loss, anemia, depression, dermatoses, diarrhea, fatigue, fragile bones, and weakness.
- **Manganese** – Important for ligament strength and preventing disc injuries (many pregnant women suffer from low back pain). Necessary for carbohydrate metabolism, and the metabolism and release of neurotransmitters, synthesis of immuno-globulins and pituitary hormones and the removal of toxic free radicals.
- **Selenium (RDA 50 - 65 mcg.)** – Important antioxidant function, helps prevent cancer and heart disease, reduces heavy metal toxicity, may decrease asthma symptoms. Converts thyroid hormone to its active form.
- **Molybdenum (no RDA, safe/adequate dosages are 75-250 mcg.)** – an important trace mineral for metabolizing odors and sulfites. Deficiency can cause allergies to perfume, cigarette smoke, etc. The sensitivity to foods at salad bars containing sulfites is also caused by this deficiency.
- **Chromium (RDA 50-200 mcg.)** – Improves glucose tolerance in both diabetics and hypoglycemics. Reduces total serum cholesterol while increasing HDL.
- **Inositol** – Improves fat metabolism.
- **Quercetin** – An important bioflavonoid with valuable anti-inflammatory and allergy-inhibiting properties. Protects against breast cancer and is also anti-viral.

ANTIOXIDANTS

This is an area of nutrition that has literally exploded in knowledge during the past decade. Antioxidants are a category of compounds that are considered our "human rust prevention." They protect our cells from aging, chemical damage and oxidation.

An example of oxidation is when you peel an apple or banana and it turns brown, that is oxidation, due to exposure to air. When you soak banana or apple slices in lemon juice to prevent them from turning brown, this is employing an "antioxidant." The lemon juice has vitamin C which is just one of many known antioxidants.

Many people are aware of the role antioxidants play in cancer prevention and slowing down the aging process. The varying degrees of skin wrinkles as we approach middle age are a reflection of our body's antioxidant function. Some of the other conditions associated with excessive oxidation include arthritis, cataracts, macular degeneration, stroke, hypoglycemia, muscle fatigue, fibromyalgia, epilepsy, Huntington's, Alzheimer's, and Parkinson's diseases, multiple sclerosis, and ALS (Lou Gehrig's disease). No wonder a recent survey of neurologists found that seventy percent of them were taking antioxidants!

Antioxidants work by neutralizing the destructive action of free radicals, which are molecules lacking an electron. Free radicals are unstable molecules that attack your cells, tearing through the cell membranes and reacting with your RNA, DNA, proteins and enzymes. These attacks, known as oxidative stress, are capable of causing cells to lose their structure and function and can eventually disable or kill the cell.

Our bodies' antioxidant systems can become overwhelmed by pollution, infection, smoking, poor diet, medications, excessive exercise and alcohol, to name a few. Antioxidants come from vitamins, minerals, enzymes and the phytonutrients found in herbs and vine-ripened fruits and vegetables.

Some antioxidants are fat-soluble and some are water-soluble. A good antioxidant formula should have some of both in order to quench the many free radicals that affect our various organs and tissues. Unfortunately, some of the antioxidant formulas on the market offer nothing more than vitamins A, C and E.

Following is an explanation of the various ingredients found in the antioxidant formula I use in my practice (**Oxygenics**™ by **Metagenics**). Some of these items were discussed prior in the prenatal sections so I have mentioned only additional information about their antioxidant role here.

You will note that the majority of antioxidant ingredients involve liver function. Because optimal nutrient status in the liver is so important for proper detoxification and cancer prevention I have devoted an entire chapter to its function. (See *Day 25-Love Your Liver*).

ANTIOXIDANT INGREDIENTS OF OXYGENICS™

- **N-acetylcysteine (NAC)** helps repair oxidative damage to tissues.
- **Manganese** is used by an important antioxidant enzyme called superoxide dismutase inside the mitochondria of our cells. The mitochondria are where we produce energy for our muscles.
- **Superoxide dismutase (SOD) precursor complex (zinc, copper, and manganase). SOD** is a key oxidative enzyme that converts the superoxide free radical into hydrogen peroxide.
- **Selenium** works in conjunction with vitamin E and helps liver detoxification.
- **Beta-carotene (as mixed carotenoids)** helps with liver detoxification.
- **Vitamin C** strengthens blood vessels and helps with liver detoxification.
- **Vitamin E** helps with liver detoxification.
- **Zinc** helps with liver detoxification.
- **Milk thistle seed extract (Silymarin)** is one of the most potent liver antioxidants and promotes liver regeneration.
- **Grape seed extract** is a bioflavonoid that helps with liver detoxification. As a free radical scavenger it is fifty times more powerful than vitamin E and twenty times more than vitamin C.
- **Glutathione** neutralizes the hydroxyl and superoxide radicals, hydrogen peroxide and lipid peroxides. It is a major antioxidant found inside the mitochondrion to protect energy production. It can also inhibit pro-inflammatory cytokines such as tumor necrosis factor. It has anti-carcinogenic effects and binds xenobiotics (toxic chemicals) and toxic metals. Glutathione has been shown to decrease during the aging process.
- **Lipoic acid** neutralizes the hydroxyl radical and hydrogen peroxide. It is a sulfur-containing organic acid that protects the mitochondrial membranes by interacting with vitamin C and glutathione to aid in the recycling of vitamin E. It is helpful for neurotoxicity, nerve degeneration, radiation injury and the reduction of heavy metal toxicity. It is also important for the regulation of insulin and blood sugar. It lengthens cell life, fights infection, increases energy and detoxifies the body.
- **Coenzyme Q-10** neutralizes hydrogen peroxide and lipid peroxides. It provides antioxidant support for the mitochondria against nitric oxide. It is important in cases of muscle weakness and decreased nerve conduction.
- **L-carnitine** helps deliver fats into the mitochondrion for energy production. It aids in function of the cardiovascular system, liver and muscles.

ESSENTIAL FATTY ACIDS

Essential fatty acids (EFA's) comprise some of the most important nutrients in the human diet. EFA's are more powerful than the calorie for promoting energy, fat loss and regeneration. They help control inflammation, allow the immune system to repair and protect itself, help produce hormones and provide critical components of the brain and nervous system. The brain has a very high fat content, and all of our nerves are lined with fat.

For these reasons, the number of diseases related to EFA imbalances and deficiencies is ***enormous***. These include pain and inflammatory disorders like arthritis and fibromyalgia, cardiovascular diseases, hormonal dysfunction, mental and behavioral disorders (including ADD and depression), and premature senility.

EFA's are also the primary constituent of our skin and can affect such conditions as dermatitis, hair loss, brittle nails, eczema, coarse, dry hair and also frequent infections. We will discuss fats more thoroughly in the *Day 23--Good Fats, "Bad Fats", HORRIBLE Fats* chapter.

SIGNS AND SYMPTOMS OF ESSENTIAL FATTY ACID DEFICIENCY:	
• Fatigue	• Hypertension
• Dry skin and hair	• Joint pain
• Pain and inflammation	• Poor memory & concentration
• Infertility	• Dry mucous membranes
• Menstrual cramps and irregularity	• Poor cognitive development in childhood
• Immune deficiency	• Insulin dysregulation
• Depression	• Poor vision
• Angina	• Blood clots, strokes

Since most Americans get ample supplies of omega-6 fats (corn oil, safflower, etc.) and omega-9 oils (olive oil) in their diets, we frequently have to supplement with omega-3 oils (fish oils, walnuts, flax seed). Our bodies need four times more omega-3 oils than omega-6 oils.

EPA/DHA or just EPA by itself in cod liver oil is the most common form of supplementation. Some vegetarians prefer to use flax seed oil, but many people are lacking an enzyme to convert it to its active form. DHA is also being given to chickens to produce DHA enriched eggs. (Note that DHA is not the same as DHEA, which is an adrenal hormone).

FOOD FOR THE BRAIN

DHA is very important to the developing fetus and infant. The human brain develops rapidly during the late stages of fetal development and early infancy. The DHA content of the fetal brain increases three to five times during the final trimester of pregnancy and triples during the first twelve weeks of life. Premature infants and those who are not breastfed are at increased risk of DHA deficiency. Inadequate levels of DHA are associated with a lower IQ in children.

Normal development of the retina and the visual cortex also depends on adequate DHA levels during the final months of pregnancy and the first six months of infancy. A child with poor vision was probably deficient in DHA during that period.

For several years now, the **World Health Organization** has been pushing developed countries to include DHA in infant baby formula. Over sixty countries have complied with this request but the United States still does not.

To help nudge our country to act more quickly there is a group of physicians trying to gain support for this cause known as "**Pregnant Doctors for DHA**."

Low DHA is also linked with certain behavioral and neurologic conditions associated with aging such as dementia, depression, memory loss, and visual problems. It may also play a role in attention-deficit/hyperactivity disorder (ADHD).

One of the first signs of EPA/DHA deficiency is a decreased ability to concentrate. This is also one of the first signs of depression. Many patients have told me their depression started in childhood. A November 30, 1999 article in **USA Today** stated "at least 500,000 children and teens in the USA are taking antidepressants. Some experts say it is considerably more and growing rapidly. **The American Academy of Child and Adolescent Psychiatry** puts the number of 'significantly' depressed children and teens at five percent, or 3.4 million youngsters."

Children who develop depression are three to four times more likely than peers to have drug or alcohol problems by their mid-20s a **Yale Medical** study shows. Suicide rates for children and teens have tripled from 1962 to 1995. Nearly one out of ten kids who develop major depression before puberty goes on to commit suicide.

Omega-3 fat supplementation should be considered for both children and adults as a means of preventing depresion and suicide. Since small children can not tolerate pills very well, perhaps we need to return to the days when children were given a dose of cod liver oil a couple of times per week. Most of the EPA/DHA pills on the market are too big for small children to swallow.

EPA/DHA supplementation should also be considered during pregnancy. Since many people are deficient in these oils, we should assume that pregnant women are also deficient. The mother and baby both need these important oils. Since omega-3 fats are noted for their ability to keep blood platelets from sticking together, this may be an important nutrient to prevent blood clots and strokes. Perhaps adequate levels of these brain-nourishing oils would also prevent post-partum depression.

Please note that EPA/DHA should not be taken with dinner. These oils nourish the brain so well that it may wake you up at night with too many creative ideas. I always recommend they be taken ten minutes before breakfast and lunch. Having your meal push these capsules down prevents you from burping the fishy taste. These oils are never combined with a multivitamin so they always need separate packaging. **Metagenics** tests their EPA/DHA for heavy metal contamination and rancidity. They also put a small amount of vitamin E in every capsule to prevent the oil's oxidation. It is recommended that bottles be refrigerated after opening to keep it fresh longer.

Perhaps you can now appreciate why I consider these categories of nutritional supplements, "The Big 3," so important. It is imperative to have a wide range of nutrients supplied every day to overcome depletion, reduce toxicity and better manage your stress. Modern nutrition research has found that every one of these nutrients plays a vital role in our health. Taking good quality nutrients that are properly combined can help you use fewer supplements with better results.

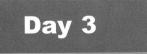
Day 3

"Obstacles are those frightful things you see
when you take your eyes off your goals."

— Unknown

Food & Activity Diary

Keeping a Food and Activity Diary can be one of your most valuable learning tools for making diet and lifestyle changes. It will raise your awareness of how well you are making changes toward rebuilding your health and vitality. Writing everything down is helpful to realize just how much flour, sugar, soda, coffee and unhealthy snacks and desserts you are consuming. This is a valuable exercise to make you more accountable for what you are putting into your mouth and how much recreation and exercise time you are allocating.

Take notice how you feel both physically and emotionally on the same day or next day after consuming foods or beverages that may not be the best for you. I once had a patient who was bothered *daily* by feelings of suicide (he was also under the care of a psychiatrist). On his first appointment I asked him to decrease his intake of dairy and wheat. To my amazement, one week later he came in and announced that he had only felt suicidal one day. When we looked at his diet chart I noticed he had eaten wheat on three days but dairy only once. The bad feelings came the day after consuming dairy. I asked him to continue observing this and it happened each time he had consumed foods containing dairy such as pizza or ice cream.

When I consume excessive quantities of chocolate I develop bizarre feelings of self-hatred and ideas that I am a failure. Since I choose not to operate my life with those feelings, I consume chocolate very rarely and in small amounts. It is just not worth it to feel that way.

These Food and Activity charts will be found throughout the book. I wanted to give you frequent reminders because this is one of the most important activities in the entire book. In future chapters you may also want to keep track of your pulse rate, breathing exercises and meditations.

When you finish the book, look back at your early charts to see how many changes you have made and how different you feel as a result of these changes. You may want to copy one of these charts and keep a health journal for a longer period of time.

"Enlightenment must come little by little-
otherwise it would overwhelm."
— Idries Shah

3 DAY FOOD & ACTIVITY DIARY

	Date:	Date:	Date:
Morning Meal Time:			
Snack			
Noon Meal Time:			
Snack			
Evening Meal Time:			
Snack			
Symptoms (Physical & Emotional)			
Exercise Type & Duration			

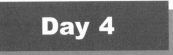

Day 4

"We are living in a world today where lemonade is made from artificial flavors and furniture polish is made from real lemons."

— Alfred E. Newman

If God Didn't Make It, Don't Eat It

One of the most controversial aspects of our food products is the use of additives, preservatives, dyes, etc. It is overwhelming to even consider all the different chemicals in our foods and what effects they may be having on our bodies. To make the decision a little easier I developed the slogan, "If God didn't make it, don't eat it."

Some nutrition experts have made the recommendation to shop the perimeter of the grocery store (meats and produce) and avoid the aisles. Just consider how many food products are sold today that were not available thirty to fifty years ago. Soda pop, which is just a concoction of sugar and chemicals, is almost popular enough to be proclaimed our national beverage. It is certainly one of our major exports!

On October 25, 1999, the nonprofit **Center for Science in the Public Interest**, issued a review of two dozen scientific studies which contend that food dyes and certain foods can adversely affect children's behavior. Their thirty-two-page report titled ***"Diet, ADHD, and Behavior,"*** charges that federal agencies, professional organizations, and the food industry ignore the growing evidence that diet affects behavior. Most of the studies focused on the effects of milk, corn, sugary breakfast cereals, cupcakes and candies. Some studies linked behavior problems to the ingredients in toothpaste, drugs and children's vitamins.

The report also raised concerns from a 1995 study, conducted by the federal government's **National Toxicology Program**, which found that the drug, Ritalin, caused liver tumors in mice. Ritalin (methylphenidate) is a stimulant medication that is prescribed to four million children in America each year for **Attention Deficit Disorder (ADD)** and **Attention Deficit/Hyperactivity Disorder (ADHD)**.

The book ***Seven Weeks to Sobriety***, by **Joan Mathews Larson, Ph.D.**, also raises the question of whether food additives, chemicals and dyes could be having toxic effects on the brain and contributing to poor concentration and short attention spans. She mentions that hyperactivity affects only ***one child in two thousand*** in Europe where less than twenty food additives are approved for use. In the U.S., where more than ***four thousand*** food additives are in use, hyperactivity affects ***one in four*** children.

In my practice I have helped many children who had poor attention spans, were unable to sit still and threw violent tantrums. Avoiding sugar, junk food and dairy products, eating more protein and vegetables, nutritional supplementation, and getting chiropractic care to balance the nervous system produced outstanding results for the majority of cases.

THE TOP 10 FOOD ADDITIVES TO AVOID

We are going to further explore caffeine and one of my pet peeves, trans or hydrogenated fats, in later chapters. The following are what the **Center for Science in the Public Interest** web site (**www.cspinet.org**) lists as the ten top food additives to avoid:

1. **Acesulfame K** – known commercially as **Sunette®** or **Sweet One®**, a sugar substitute sold in packets or tablets and contained in gum, dry beverage mixes, instant coffee and tea, gelatin desserts, puddings and non-dairy creamers. Tests show that it causes cancer in animals.

2. **Artificial Colorings** – The majority of these are synthetic dyes that have been under suspicion for decades as being toxic or carcinogenic. Many doctors have written books with the concern that they contribute to allergies, learning disabilities and anti-social behaviors.

3. **Aspartame** – known commercially as **Equal®** or **NutraSweet®**. This product has several problems including causing mental retardation in one out of twenty thousand babies. This product should certainly be avoided by pregnant women. In **Dr. Nancy Appleton's** book, *Lick The Sugar Habit*, she notes the methanol in aspartame is toxic to the brain and liver and could eventually exhaust the immune and endocrine systems. Thousands of consumer complaints against aspartame include dizziness, vision problems, disorientation, ear buzzing, liver enzyme elevations, loss of equilibrium, severe muscle aches, numbness of extremities, pancreas inflammation, high blood pressure and eye hemorrhages.

4. **BHA & BHT** – two related chemicals added to oil-containing foods to prevent oxidation and slow rancidity. The **International Agency for Research on Cancer**, part of the **World Health Organization**, considers BHA to be possibly carcinogenic to humans. According to the CSPI, BHT and BHA are totally unnecessary and should be phased out of our food.

5. **Caffeine** – one of the few drugs, a stimulant, added to foods. Caffeine promotes stomach acid secretion, temporarily raises blood pressure, and dilates some blood vessels while constricting others. Caffeine may also interfere with reproduction and affect developing fetuses. Experiments on lab animals link caffeine to birth defects such as cleft palates, missing fingers and toes and skull malformations.

6. **Monosodium Glutamate (MSG)** – a seasoning that enhances the flavor of protein-containing foods. Unfortunately, excessive amounts of MSG can lead to headaches, tightness in the chest, and a burning sensation in the forearms and the back of the neck. Some highly sensitive individuals react to even small amounts of MSG. Also avoid hydrolyzed vegetable protein, or HVP, which may contain MSG.

7. **Nitrite and Nitrate** – used for centuries to preserve meat. When nitrite combines with compounds called secondary amines, it forms nitrosamines, extremely powerful cancer-causing chemicals. This chemical reaction occurs most readily at the high temperatures of frying. Nitrite has long been suspected of being a cause of stomach cancer. Look for nitrite-free processed meats, some of which are frozen.

8. **Olestra®** – the fake fat recently approved by the **Food and Drug Administration** is both dangerous and unnecessary. Olestra was approved over the objection of dozens of leading scientists. The additive may be fat-free but it has a fatal side-effect: it attaches to valuable nutrients and flushes them out of the body. Some of the nutrients, called carotenoids, appear to protect us from such diseases as lung cancer, prostate cancer, heart disease, and macular degeneration. The **Harvard School of Public Health** states that "the long-term consumption of olestra snack foods might therefore result in several thousand unnecessary deaths each year from lung and prostate cancers and heart disease, and hundreds of additional cases of blindness in the elderly due to macular degeneration. In addition to contributing to disease, olestra causes diarrhea and other serious gastrointestinal problems, even at low doses."

9. **Saccharin** – Several studies in the 1970's linked saccharin with cancer in laboratory animals. Sweetener packets and cans of saccharin-containing diet drinks bear warning labels: "Use of this product may be hazardous to your health. This product contains saccharine, which has been determined to cause cancer in laboratory animals." CSPI asks, "Why not heed the warning? "

10. **Sulfites** – a class of chemicals that can keep cut fruits and vegetables looking fresh. Sulfites prevent discoloration in apricots, raisins, and other dried fruits; control "black spot" in freshly caught shrimp; and prevent discoloration, bacterial growth and fermentation in wine. Until the early 1980's they were considered safe, but CSPI and the FDA identified at least a dozen fatalities linked to sulfites, all among asthmatics. In 1985, Congress finally forced the FDA to ban sulfites from most fruits and vegetables. The ban does not cover fresh-cut potatoes, dried fruits and wine.

ADD UP YOUR TYPICAL "EXTRACURRICULAR" EXPENDITURES

Over the years, I have heard many people declare that they cannot possibly afford organic vegetables, better cuts of meats, a water purifier or nutritional supplements. Supplementing with the "Big 3" presently costs only $2 per day. Many people spend more than that on just a single cup of coffee. When we become aware of how much money we already waste on foods, beverages, junk foods, etc. that detract from our health, we have to wonder why we begrudge spending just a couple of dollars per day on things that protect our health. Even people who smoke or drink alcohol daily often do not take vitamins to prevent the well-known deficiencies associated with these habits.

TODAY'S ACTIVITY

The following is a chart to help you see what you presently spend on products that are not the most desirable for your health. Take a good look at what you spend for an entire week and decide if you want to explore other plans with your money.

	Sun.	Mon.	Tues.	Wed.	Thurs.	Fri.	Sat.	Total
candy/gum								
bakery								
snack cakes								
chips/dips								
fast food								
tobacco								
soda pop								
caffeine								
alcohol								
TV dinners								
ice cream								
other								

"The beginning of a habit is like an invisible thread, but every time we repeat the act we strengthen the strand, add to it another filament, until it becomes a great cable and binds us irrevocably, thought and act."
— Orison Sweet Marden

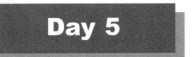

**"You will come to know
that what appears today to be a sacrifice
will prove instead to be the greatest investment
that you will ever make."**

—Gorden B. Hinkley

The Sugar Blues

I can remember growing up as a child in the 50's during the "Sugar is Instant Energy" campaign. Media advertising extolled the virtues of sugar for providing energy. I recall opening up sugar packets in restaurants and pouring them into my mouth, because I wanted to have more energy. I can also remember other times when I was so hypoglycemic upon waking that I would literally crawl to the bread box to get some white bread to increase my blood sugar.

Imagine my dismay when I found out, two decades later, this whole campaign was orchestrated by the sugar industry. According to the book, *Sugar Blues,* by **William Dufty**, various sugar-related companies paid a quarter of a million dollars to an Ivy League University's nutrition program in exchange for developing favorable research projects that extolled the virtues of sugar.

To this day, when I give health seminars and suggest eliminating *all* refined sugars and carbohydrates from the daily diet, I get worried questions from people who have been led to believe that *some amount* of sugar is *mandatory* for good health; as though it has a place of honor on top of the **USDA's** food pyramid.

Sugar has a huge psychological impact on our society. Sugar is "love" and everyone wants more love in their lives. One patient once told me, "Sugar is my best friend." Sugar is used as a reward from earliest childhood and continues throughout life as a way to celebrate or medicate yourself when you are feeling good or bad. Candy and cookies are common gifts among friends.

Sugar is the ultimate party food and source of comfort . Every special occasion or holiday has a significant dessert or treat associated with it – birthday, wedding and anniversary cakes, Valentine's chocolates, Easter jellybeans, Halloween candy, Thanksgiving pies, Christmas cookies and gingerbread houses.

The only problem is, our hedonistic society has made every day a party! We cannot wait for the next party to reward ourselves with sugar. We have to put chocolate in our breakfast cereals and milk. We drink soda pop or a sweet beverage with every meal. We eat cookies between meals and ice cream or other desserts every night after dinner.

One of the most common causes of fatigue (and gaining weight and body fat) is consuming too many low quality carbohydrates, such as sugar and refined flours. The more refined the carbohydrates, the worse your fatigue.

When I look at patients' diet and activity charts, I see multiple meals where the predominant foods at each meal are made from flour and/or sugar. It is not unusual for me to count eight to twelve servings of refined carbohydrates per day on these charts.

Breakfast is usually toast, pancakes, waffles, toaster pastries, breakfast cereals, donuts, bagels, granola bars, etc. Lunch, snacks and dinner are loaded with sandwiches, noodles, macaroni, pasta, tortillas, pizza, crackers, cookies, pies, cakes, and so forth. Add to that the popular sources of sugar, soda pop (ten teaspoons of sugar per can), candy bars, alcohol, "diet" shakes (often thirty-five percent sugar), juices, ice cream and milk shakes, and you can see why diabetes has exploded in the past decade. It is not unusual for people to consume entire liters of soda at one sitting.

SUGAR WHERE YOU LEAST EXPECT IT

Sugar is added to just about everything (including salt). You can find sugar on labels by looking for words ending in "ose." Sucrose, fructose, dextrose, glucose, maltose, levulose, galactose and lactose are all sugars. In addition, there are corn sweeteners, corn syrup, honey, turbinado sugar, molasses, maple sugar, dextrine, barley malt and rice syrup.

Some products, like granola bars, have as many as ten forms of sugar. **Dr. Nancy Appleton**, in her 1996 book, ***Lick the Sugar Habit***, offers the following list of hidden sugars:

- Many meat packers feed sugar to animals prior to slaughter. This improves the flavor and color of cured meat.
- Sugar (in the form of corn syrup and dehydrated molasses) is often added to hamburgers sold in restaurants to reduce shrinkage.
- The breading on many prepared foods contains sugar.
- Before salmon is canned, it is often glazed with a sugar solution.
- Some fast-food restaurants sell poultry that has been injected with a flavorful honey solution.
- Sugar is used in the processing of luncheon meats, bacon, and canned meats.
- Sugar is found in bouillon cubes and dry-roasted nuts.
- Sugar is found in beer, wine, and other alcoholic beverages. Champagne and cordials have an unusually high sugar content.
- Sugar is often added to the syrup in canned fruits.
- Peanut butter and many dry cereals (even corn flakes) contain sugar.
- Almost half the calories found in most commercial ketchups come from sugar.
- Over ninety percent of the calories found in the average can of cranberry sauce come from sugar.
- Over 1,500 drugs contain hidden cornstarch or lactose (milk sugar). The law allows lactose and cornstarch to be labeled as "inert substances," and their presence may be concealed even from your doctor or pharmacist.

TODAY'S ACTIVITY

Look over your Diet and Activity chart and circle or highlight all foods
that are likely to contain sugar.

SUGAR AND DIABETES

Twenty years ago, doctors were trained to start looking for type 2 (adult-onset) diabetes in someone who fit the profile of the "three F's:" Female, Fat and Forty. On September 4, 2000, **Newsweek** magazine printed a feature story on diabetes, which stated some very grim facts about the new prevalence of this disease. There has been a dramatic rise in diabetes among people in their thirties and even in children, making the term "adult-onset" diabetes **obsolete**.

Type 2 diabetes differs from type 1 (juvenile) diabetes in that it increases the risk of heart disease several-fold. A similar increased risk of stroke occurs in type 2 diabetics versus non-diabetics. **The most important reason to identify diabetes is to reduce cardiovascular diseases and deaths.** Early intervention in the nutrition habits of people who are starting to develop early insulin resistance is very important.

During the 1990's, there was an unprecedented sixty percent increase in the number of overweight Americans. In 1991, only seven states had obesity rates over fifteen percent. By 1998, only five states **did not**. According to the **Centers for Disease Control**, each year, an estimated 300,000 Americans die of causes related to obesity.

The "low-fat/no-fat" diet fads of the 1990's were obviously a dismal failure. People heartily consumed any food that advertised low-fat/no-fat and proceeded to gain more weight than ever. Unfortunately, they discovered the majority of excess carbohydrate gets converted into fat. This is where we get the term "beer belly" when describing weight gain among heavy drinkers.

I was thrilled when the book, **Sugar Busters!**™, by **Steward, Bethea, Andrews**, and **Balart**, became popular in 1998. It seemed like the first time medical doctors were waging a well-publicized war against sugar. In typical fashion, many of their peers ridiculed this valuable information, despite the evidence this approach reversed serious disease. This reminds me of the opening paragraph, written by one of my first nutrition mentors, in his groundbreaking book, **Psychodietetics:**

> "Any important 'new idea' has to go through three stages:
> first ridicule, then discussion, and finally, general acceptance.
> — Emanuel Cheraskin, M.D., D.M.D.

Dr. Cheraskin's book, *Psychodietetics*, co-written in 1974, with **Dr. W.M. Ringsdorf, Jr.** and **Arline Brecher**, described how blood sugar problems, associated with a refined foods diet, can lead to serious brain dysfunction and mental illnesses. Their book outlines how better nourishment can lead to recovery or improvement of mental illnesses. Unfortunately, the writers of *Psychodietetics* were way ahead of their time. Nutrition therapies are still not commonly used in the treatment of these disorders.

BLOOD SUGAR REGULATION

Understanding blood sugar is the key to maintaining good health and abundant energy. When your carbohydrate intake is excessive or too refined (sugar, alcohol, white flour, etc.), your body releases more insulin than normal to counter the rapid rise in blood sugar. Excessive insulin secretion causes your blood sugar to drop too low. This rebound of hypoglycemia causes you to experience hunger (cravings), fatigue, mental confusion and depression.

In normal individuals, blood sugar levels do not vary widely due to the complimentary actions of insulin and glucagon, both secreted by the pancreas. Insulin prevents blood sugar from rising too high and glucagon prevents it from falling too low. Glucagon secretion is stimulated by hypoglycemia, fasting, and also by the ingestion of a protein-rich meal.

Glucagon secretion is very important to optimal health and weight control, because it allows us to utilize fat as energy. Think of it as the "action" hormone. It improves energy and endurance, increases mental clarity and alertness and decreases hunger. Your food cravings naturally disappear and your body can start to use stored fat as energy. This helps decrease your body fat percentage.

Insulin is the "storage" hormone that promotes the storage of sugar, as glycogen, in both the liver and muscle. It also promotes the storage of protein in muscle and stores fat in our fat cells, as triglycerides. There is only a limited area in our bodies for glycogen storage so many carbohydrates are converted to fats for storage. Excessive sugar and refined carbohydrates are the major culprits for elevated triglycerides on your lab tests.

Insulin prevents the breakdown of glycogen and triglycerides. Even low levels of circulating insulin will prevent fat breakdown. Insulin promotes fat *deposition*. This is why you will not lose weight when insulin levels are constantly elevated by frequent carbohydrate consumption. Eating sugars and flour products all day long at meals and snacks causes continuous insulin elevation. This results in frequent sugar cravings and sets your body up for instant gratification to balance the blood sugar. It is much more efficient to have your body "trained" to release glucagon as a way to utilize fat for energy in between meals.

Insulin also favors inflammatory processes that can cause heart disease and arthritis. Glucagon promotes healing and repair processes and encourages anti-inflammatory pathways. This helps reverse chronic pain and inflammation problems.

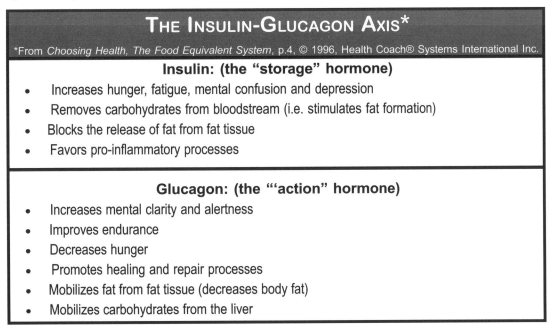

THE INSULIN-GLUCAGON AXIS*

*From *Choosing Health, The Food Equivalent System*, p.4, © 1996, Health Coach® Systems International Inc.

Insulin: (the "storage" hormone)

- Increases hunger, fatigue, mental confusion and depression
- Removes carbohydrates from bloodstream (i.e. stimulates fat formation)
- Blocks the release of fat from fat tissue
- Favors pro-inflammatory processes

Glucagon: (the "'action" hormone)

- Increases mental clarity and alertness
- Improves endurance
- Decreases hunger
- Promotes healing and repair processes
- Mobilizes fat from fat tissue (decreases body fat)
- Mobilizes carbohydrates from the liver

One of the most powerful ways to restore your energy and vitality is to restore balance to insulin and glucagon. This can be done by correcting protein to carbohydrate ratios at ***each meal*** and choosing higher quality carbohydrates. Sugar will ***never*** correct hypoglycemia. Only by avoiding refined carbohydrates and increasing protein, vegetables, and whole grains, will you bring blood sugar under control.

SYNDROME X

Syndrome X is a term first described by **Dr. G.M. Reaven** to describe a constellation of symptoms revolving around insulin resistance. Insulin resistance is a condition of decreased responsiveness to insulin by fat cells, liver cells and muscle cells. This requires much higher levels of insulin secretion to handle blood sugar levels.

SYNDROME X IS PRESENT WHEN YOU HAVE TWO OR MORE OF THE FOLLOWING CONDITIONS:

- Insulin resistance with resulting elevated insulin levels
- Elevated lipids - triglycerides >200 and HDL <35
- Obesity or elevated body fat
- Coronary artery disease
- High blood pressure >145/90
- Elevations of high sensitivity C Reactive Protein (CRP) – a sign of inflammation

Native Americans and Asians are genetically predisposed to develop insulin resistance. The **Pima Indians** of Arizona have had an explosion of type 2 diabetes in their culture. In the 1930's, there was no diabetes among the Pimas. In the 1990's, seventy percent were diabetic.

Obesity is the most common result of insulin resistance. ***Insulin resistance causes obesity, not vice versa.*** The type of obesity most associated with blood sugar problems is the "apple shape," where the waist becomes larger than the hips. However, measuring body fat sometimes identifies a new health classification of patients known as **MONW**, which stands for ***"metabolically obese, normal weight."*** This patient does not look overweight but their body fat is increasing and their lean muscle mass is decreasing, due to insulin imbalances. In my practice, I measure body fat on every new patient to identify early problems with insulin. Just recently, I found a body fat reading of ***fifty-eight percent*** on an obese sixteen year-old girl. I strongly urged her parent to have her tested for diabetes. Doctors need to stress early intervention on high refined-carbohydrate diets to prevent diabetes, heart disease and cancer.

HEALTHY BODY FAT RANGE		
	Under 30 yrs old	Over 30 yrs old
Male	14%-20%	17%-23%
Female	17%-24%	20%-27%

THE GLYCEMIC INDEX

In order to choose foods that will cause the least insulin secretion, you need to avoid foods with a high *"Glycemic Index."* The **glycemic index** was first published by **Dr. David Jenkins**, in a 1981 issue of the ***American Journal of Clinical Nutrition.*** The index is based on glucose, the type of sugar used by our bodies for energy, which has a score of one hundred. Foods with higher numbers (sixty to one hundred) have the most disruptive effect on insulin. The chart on the next page shows a greater variety of foods. Proteins such as meat, fish and eggs have no carbohydrate content unless they contain sugar, such as bacon, ham and sausage. Beans have very low scores, with soybean being the best. Although some fruits and vegetables have fairly high scores, green leafy vegetables are extremely low (zero to fifteen). Do not be misled by the relatively low score of sucrose. The bigger the dose taken, the greater the insulin response. A "supersize" soda can have as many as twenty to thirty teaspoons of sugar. Note how the refining process causes more disruption to blood sugar, with the following examples of rice and wheat.

RICE AND WHEAT GLYCEMIC INDEX SCORES			
Instant rice	90	White pretzels	85
Rice cakes	80	White bread and bagels	75
Rice Krispies	80	Total & Cheerios cereals	75
White rice	70	Whole-wheat crackers	65
Basmati rice	60	Special K cereal	55
Brown rice	55	Cracked-wheat bread	50
Whole rice	50	Pita bread, stone-ground	45
		All Bran, wheat grain	45

Glycemic Index of Some Common Foods

Sugars		**Grains**	
Glucose	100	Rye grain	35
Maltose	105	Barley grain	45
Honey	75	Oatmeal	55
Sucrose	60	Wild rice	55
Fructose	20	Pasta	65
Fruits		Millet	70
Grapefruit, cherries	25	Taco shells, corn meal	70
Apples, peaches, plums, oranges	40	Puffed wheat	75
Grapes, kiwi, mango	50	Corn chips, corn flakes	75
Raisins, pineapple	65	**Legumes**	
Watermelon	70	Soy beans	15
Vegetables		Lima, black, butter and kidney	30
Green peas	45	Pintos, lentils and green beans	40
Sweet potatoes	55	**Other foods**	
Potato, boiled	70	Ice cream	60
Beets	75	Milk	30
Carrots	85	Plain yogurt	15
Potato, baked	95	Nuts	15-30

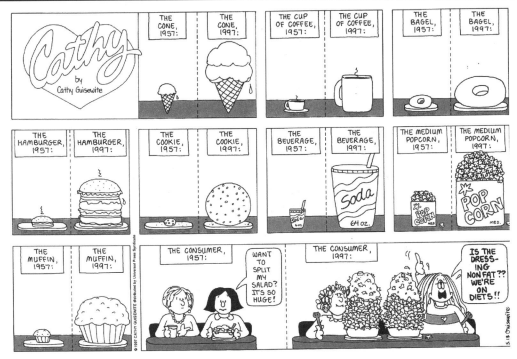

TODAY'S ACTIVITY

Determining Your Sensitivity to Insulinogenic Foods and Eating Habits

(From *Choosing Health, The Food Equivalent System*, ©1996, **Dr. Mark Percival**)

Please fill in this questionnaire to determine your relative sensitivity to insulinogenic foods and eating habits. *Please place the number in parentheses on the line for every YES answer.* Total your score at the end.

(5) _____ I have a tendency to higher blood pressure.

(5) _____ I gain weight easily, especially around my waist and have difficulty losing it.

(5) _____ I often experience mental confusion.

(5) _____ I often experience fatigue and generalized weakness.

(10) _____ I have diabetic tendencies.

(4) _____ I get tired and/or hungry in the mid-afternoon.

(5) _____ About an hour or two after eating a full meal that includes dessert, I want more of the dessert.

(3) _____ It is harder for me to control my eating for the rest of the day if I have a breakfast containing carbohydrates, than it would be if I had only coffee or nothing at all.

(4) _____ When I want to lose weight, I find it easier to not eat for most of the day than to try to eat several small diet meals.

(3) _____ Once I start eating sweets, starches, or snack foods, I often have a difficult time stopping.

(3) _____ I would rather have an ordinary meal that included dessert than a gourmet meal that did not include dessert.

(5) _____ After finishing a full meal, I sometimes feel I could go back and eat the whole meal again.

(3) _____ A meal of only meat and vegetables leaves me feeling unsatisfied.

(3) _____ If I'm feeling down, a snack of cake or cookies makes me feel better.

(3) _____ If potatoes, bread, pasta, or dessert are on the table, I will often skip eating vegetables or salad.

(4) _____ I get a sleepy, almost "drugged" feeling after eating a large meal containing bread or pasta or potatoes and dessert, whereas I feel more energetic after a meal of only meat or fish and salad.

(3) _____ I have a hard time going to sleep at times without a bedtime snack.

(3) _____ Sometimes I wake in the middle of the night and can't go back to sleep unless I eat something.

(5) _____ I get irritable if I miss a meal or mealtime is delayed.

(2) _____ At a restaurant, I almost always eat too much bread, even before the meal is served.

_____**Total**

Important note: The higher the score, the more fastidious you should be regarding your protein to carbohydrate ratios at each meal.

Scoring:

1-20   **Consume low fat/high complex carbohydrates**

25+   **Consume moderate protein, low starch**

VITAMIN AND MINERAL DEPLETION BY SUGAR

There is still a lot of misunderstanding about the quality of carbohydrates and how they affect the body. In September, 2000, an advice column, in a popular fitness magazine, stated that our bodies cannot tell the difference between the sugars in colas and orange juice. Certainly, sucrose and fructose both get converted into glucose, but the key is ***how many nutrients are spent*** during the conversion.

The lack of nutrients in sugar and white flour products is the primary danger to our health and vitality. Sugar does not have a single nutrient – ***zero*** vitamins and minerals. This is why sugar is sometimes referred to as "empty calories." White flour has about twenty-six nutrients refined out and about a dozen added back. Those nutrients added back are not even the same amount as originally present. Also, different types of white flour products, such as bread, crackers, cookies and pasta are not always fortified with the same nutrients.

Our body puts carbohydrates through a large number of metabolic reactions to convert them to energy. The major portion of this energy metabolism is known as the **Kreb's Cycle** or **Citric Acid Cycle** (see figure 5.1). In biochemistry books the reactions of this cycle are written in a circular fashion much like the face of a clock. Each metabolic conversion of sugar requires various vitamins and minerals. The primary nutrients required to fuel these many reactions include thiamin (B-1), riboflavin (B-2), niacinamide (B-3), pantothenic acid (B-5), pyridoxine (B-6), lipoic acid, manganese, biotin, magnesium, iron, sulfur, phosphorus and coenzyme Q-10.

Because sugar has no nutrients of its own to give up to this process, all of these reactions happen by using "borrowed" nutrients from your organs and tissues. If you never eat high-quality, nutrient-rich foods, these borrowed nutrients never get paid back and you become weak, tired and eventually diseased. It is similar to buying things on a credit card that you can never possibly pay back. This is why ***not even the healthiest*** of our bodies can afford to consume sugar and refined foods on a ***daily*** basis.

Eventually the nutrient storage areas become depleted and we develop "biochemical imbalances," which is another name for malnutrition. The biochemical reactions stop happening correctly because there are inadequate nutrients to drive them. This is why fatigue, depression and memory/concentration problems all happen simultaneously. Our muscles and brain become starved and the brain is the first organ to show problems. The brain is the most nutrient-dependent organ in our bodies because it tells everything else what to do.

All of the conversion steps of the **Kreb's cycle** involve various forms of organic acids. If a person has a serious deficit of certain nutrients, the next conversion does not happen and the organic acids can build up in our muscles. This excess of organic acids can result in severe fatigue and muscle pains. This can set the stage for symptoms associated with chronic fatigue syndrome and fibromyalgia. Levels of these organic acids can be measured in the urine to find disruptions in the energy metabolism. **Great Smokies Lab** has a test called the **Cellular**

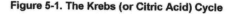

Figure 5-1. The Krebs (or Citric Acid) Cycle

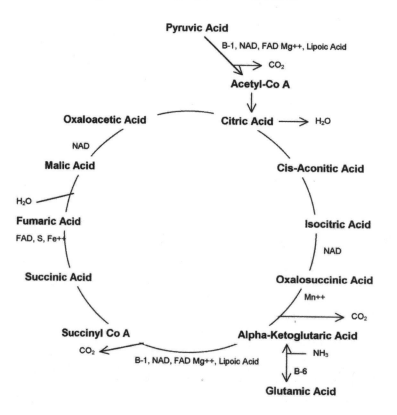

Your body cannot afford nutrient-depleted foods. Consider them very dangerous and never consume them frequently. You cannot even use small quantities of poor quality foods and expect to recover from fatigue. If you are seriously ill you may have to give up these foods for many months or even years to recover your health.

Sugar does not build your energy and vitality. It may raise your blood sugar temporarily, but it is a very poor source of fuel. It robs your energy and depletes you every time you consume it. Biochemically, you are courting disaster and one day your health will suffer when your cells become insulin resistant or your weakest organ can no longer function normally.

For many people, the weakest organ is your brain. If you combine vitamin and mineral malnutrition, with the lack of fresh fruits and vegetables, along with a deficiency in essential fatty acids, you are guaranteed to have a "biochemical imbalance" that will never be cured with Ritalin, antidepressants or psychotherapy.

We are not doing our children a favor with daily doses of sugar-laden breakfast cereals, soda pop, ice cream and candy treats! They need high quality foods to grow properly. Sugary foods and beverages and refined flours need to be relegated back to the status of "party food," and taken *out* of our daily diets.

CARBOHYDRATE CONTENT OF FRUITS AND VEGETABLES

I have found that steering people toward the lower carbohydrate fruits and vegetables is also very helpful for both blood sugar control and body fat reduction. Following, and on the next page, are lists to help you make better choices. The two columns on the left are where you should choose the majority of your foods. Eat foods from the two columns on the right only once or twice per week if you are trying to decrease your body fat.

There are nearly two times as many foods on the left side, so finding plenty of variety should not be a problem. Note that leafy vegetables, such as chard, lettuce, mustard greens, spinach, kale and collards are in the most desirable columns. These will be discussed in more detail in **Day 10 - Green Inside is Clean Inside**.

CARBOHYDRATE CLASSIFICATIONS OF VEGETABLES
(ACCORDING TO CARBOHYDRATE CONTENT)
From *Choosing Health, The Food Equivalent System*, © 1996, Dr. Mark Percival

VEGETABLES

Lowest 3 %	Lower 6%	Higher 15%	Highest 20+%
Asparagus	Beans, string	Artichokes	Beans, dried
Bean Sprouts	Beets	Oyster Plant	Beans, lima
Beet Greens	Brussels Sprouts	Parsnips	Corn
Broccoli	Chives	Peas, green	Potato, white
Cabbage	Collards	Squash	Potato, sweet
Cauliflower	Dandelion Greens	Carrots	Yams
Celery	Eggplant		
Chard, Swiss	Kale		
Cucumber	Kohlrabi		
Endive	Leeks		
Lettuce	Okra		
Mustard Greens	Onions		
Radishes	Parsley		
Spinach	Peppers, red		
	Pimento		
	Pumpkin		
	Rutabagas		
	Turnips		

CARBOHYDRATE CLASSIFICATIONS OF FRUITS
(ACCORDING TO CARBOHYDRATE CONTENT)
From *Choosing Health, The Food Equivalent System*, © 1996, Dr. Mark Percival

FRUITS			
Lowest 3%	**Lower** 6%	**Higher** 15%	**Highest** 20+%
Cantaloupe	Apricots (fresh only)	Apples	Bananas
Rhubarb	Blackberries	Blueberries	Figs
Strawberries	Cranberries	Cherries	Prunes
Watermelon	Grapefruit	Grapes	Any dried fruits
Melons	Guava	Kumquats	
Tomatoes	Melons	Loganberries	
	Lemons	Mangoes	
	Limes	Mulberries	
	Oranges	Pears	
	Papayas	Pineapples (fresh)	
	Peaches	Pomegranates	
	Plums		
	Raspberries		
	Tangerines		
	Kiwis		

SUGAR'S ROLE IN INFECTIONS

Sugar not only weakens our organs and tissues, it also feeds bad germs and sets the stage for infections and chronic ill health. Become aware that there are always "flu epidemics" within two weeks of every major "high sugar holiday." Watch this phenomenon kick into gear right after Halloween and continue until after Easter.

Observe who "catches" the flu and how long they are ill. For myself, drinking a full glass of eggnog is a guaranteed sinus infection. I love the flavor but I can only afford small doses if I want to stay healthy over the holidays. The only time I get a cold is when I have had a significant emotional stress. I typically do not "catch" other people's germs. I am usually not sick enough to miss work and the worst is over within forty-eight hours. I have seen many patients who were sick for four to six *weeks*.

Most *healthy* people do not need flu shots. We need to remind ourselves that by consuming sugary foods we are throwing a party for bad germs that weaken our immunity. We all harbor "bad germs" in our bodies. They are not always the fearsome bad guys we make them out to be. They are more likely to take over and make us ill when we weaken our immunity and strengthen them with a feast of sweets.

Dr. Emanuel Cheraskin did nutritional research for many years at the **University of Alabama**. He published over eight hundred articles and books. In the 1970's he did an experiment that tested the effectiveness of human white blood cells after various size doses of sugar. His research found that the higher the dose of sugar, the fewer germs a white blood cell was able to destroy per hour. I credit my avoidance of sugar as the primary reason I no longer "catch" infections.

Another form of sugar that is coming under increased scrutiny is milk sugar or lactose. Epidemiological studies are showing that this is one of the more inflammatory forms of sugar and may have as much correlation with the development of heart disease as the fat content of milk. Skim, one percent, and two percent milk all have similar amounts of lactose. Plain yogurt products have most of the lactose digested and would be the preferred form of dairy products.

Eliminating sugar foods is also very important when trying to correct an overabundance of yeast and other germs that live in the body (see *Day 13--What's Bugging You?"* and *Day 24--The 4 R Program*). In addition to eliminating those foods already discussed, I recommend the avoidance of all alcohol and fruit juices and consume a maximum of one fruit per day.

GLUCOSE TOLERANCE FACTOR

It has been known for several decades that chromium is involved with glucose and fat metabolism. Chromium improves insulin resistance and was first given the name "glucose tolerance factor" when it was discovered to help blood sugar in 1955. However, most diabetic patients I have worked with have never been taught the importance of chromium by their doctor or dietician.

Chromium picolinate was the most commonly used form of chromium until it was suspected of having side effects. The preferred form used today is chromium dinicotinate or dinicotinate glycinate. Chromium prevents sticky plaquing in arteries much the same way a chromium surface prevents anything from sticking to it. Vanadium is another trace mineral that works with chromium for blood sugar metabolism and is found in many multivitamin/mineral and blood sugar balancing formulas.

NEW ADVANCES IN BLOOD SUGAR CONTROL

UltraGlycemX™ is a new insulin-stabilizing medical food released by **Dr. Jeffrey Bland**, of the **Institute of Functional Medicine** in Spring, 2000. It was researched and formulated for over two years before being released. **UltraGlycemX™** is designed to provide nutritional support to individuals who are suspected of having insulin dysregulation. It comes with a thirty-four-page patient guide to teach how to combine this beverage with a low-glycemic, high-fiber dietary program. **UltraGlycemX™** is distributed by **Metagenics** (see Resources).

UltraGlycemX™ is helpful for those with type 2 diabetes, hypoglycemia, Syndrome X, obesity, hypertension, and high triglycerides. It combines soy protein, several nutrients and a patented starch that is able to moderate blood glucose and insulin levels. In just six months, this formula has become one of the most popular nutritional products in our office. It makes an ideal choice for adding protein to breakfast and helps restore energy and blood sugar stability faster than anything we have used previously. In addition, we have seen noticeable reductions in body fat and weight in those who have used it for two months or more, along with regular exercise.

ARTIFICIAL SWEETENERS

In the previous chapter, I discussed the toxicity issues with artificial sweeteners. In my opinion, the risks are not worth it. I would rather someone use sugar than an artificial sweetener. I have seen many patients over the years who were not willing to give up their diet sodas, etc., despite the fact that they had many of the health problems attributed to these chemicals. Artificial sweeteners have never been proven to cause weight loss. Since ninety percent of diabetics suffer vision problems, it makes no sense to ingest a product that could also have a negative impact on vision.

My autoimmune condition was triggered by eight months of formaldehyde exposure. Since formaldehyde is a toxic by-product associated with aspartame, this is certainly not something I can endorse.

When I am using sweeteners for baking purposes, I use rice bran syrup, which has a consistency similar to honey; or barley malt, which is more like a dark corn syrup. Neither of these products have caused blood sugar problems for me.

Sugar is the ultimate depleter of nutrients. Consider it to be as lowly as a thief. My most important message in this chapter is: ***You will never overcome fatigue and poor health unless you no longer consume nutrient-depleted foods on a daily basis.***

"The quality of a person's life is in direct proportion to their commitment to excellence."
— Vince Lombardi

"Red meat is not bad for you.
Now blue-green meat, that's bad for you!"
—Tommy Smothers

Are You Getting Enough Protein?

Sometimes when I am looking over clients' diet charts they remind me of the old Wendy's hamburger commercials, "Where's the beef?" Some of their diets are nearly devoid of protein and they wonder why they feel exhausted. When the body is starved of protein or is under stress, it will start consuming your lean muscle mass and cause you to feel very weak and exhausted. The medical term for this is "sarcopenia" and it is becoming more common in today's "carbo-crazed" culture. Doctors can identify this problem early on if they routinely measure hand-grip strength and body fat on their patients.

Protein is required for the growth, maintenance and repair of all body tissues. It is also needed to make enzymes and hormones that regulate body processes. Some proteins transport oxygen, while others form antibodies used by the immune system. Vitamins and minerals are bound to specific protein carriers for transport. Protein is also necessary for blood clotting and fluid balance. Not very much happens in the body without protein!

It has been said that an ideal portion of meat is about the size of a deck of cards. Some people eat two or three times that size and then have no appetite left for the five servings of vegetables needed per day. One of the ways I suggest people get more vegetables, along with their protein, is to eat soups or stir-fry meals (where you cook about four or five vegetables along with protein). I suggest starting with onions, and then add a combination of any of the following: celery, carrots, yellow squash, zucchini, broccoli, cabbages, snow peas, etc. You can add garlic, ginger or sesame seeds for more flavor. These are very quick meals that take only about fifteen minutes to prepare.

Vegetarianism can also pose a problem to adequate protein intake. The problem I see frequently with vegetarians, is that the many of their meals are based on low quality starches such as pizza, bread, pasta, and white rice. This is not adequate protein! Making the commitment to eat vegetarian requires that you plan meals carefully and combine high quality bean products with whole grains.

I put many clients on soy protein drinks to raise their levels of protein intake. Teenagers, athletes and the elderly are especially vulnerable to inadequate protein intake. Protein deficiency can be as detrimental to our health as vitamin and mineral deficiencies.

Our bodies use twenty to thirty grams of protein each day. To prevent protein loss, it is recommended we consume sixty to seventy-five grams of protein daily. A daily protein requirement of 0.8 grams per kilogram (one kilogram equals 2.2 pounds) body weight has been established for adults in the U.S. That calculates to fifty-five grams of protein per day for a person who weighs 150 pounds.

EACH OF THE FOLLOWING REPRESENTS APPROXIMATELY 15 GRAMS OF QUALITY PROTEIN:

From *Choosing Health, The Food Equivalent System*, © 1996, Health Coach Systems International, Inc.

Whey protein, "Perfect Protein"	¾ scoop
Whole eggs	2 large
Dairy: low fat cottage cheese	½ cup
low fat, low lactose yogurt	1 cup
Lean meat (organic is best)	2 oz.
Poultry (free range, drug free)	2 oz.
Wild game	2 oz.
Legumes: beans, tofu, lentils	6 oz.
Soy protein powder	1 oz.
Metagenics UltraMeal®, UltraGlycemX™	2 scoops
Fresh cold-water fish:	
Salmon, mackerel, trout, etc.	3 oz.
Tuna (water packed)	2 oz.
Sardines (best in sardine oil)	2 oz.

AMINO ACIDS

The basic structural unit of protein is the amino acid. Protein synthesis requires all of the necessary amino acids to be available in appropriate ratios. Of the twenty amino acids most utilized in our bodies, nine are classified *"essential"* because the body cannot synthesize them or provide them in sufficient quantities.

Dietary proteins differ in quality and therefore differ in their ability to be utilized in the body. A dietary protein that contains all of the essential amino acids in sufficient quantity and ratio is called a ***complete protein*** (high quality). When a dietary protein has a different or deficient ratio of amino acids compared to body proteins it is called an ***incomplete protein***.

Biologic Value (**BV**) is a measurement of how well proteins are utilized by the body. Animal proteins such as eggs, milk, meat, and fish are high BV, complete proteins. Vegetable proteins such as grains, legumes, nuts, and seeds are incomplete proteins and thus have a lower BV. Vegetarians can combine the lower BV proteins to make better quality mixtures of amino acids and therefore make their meal contain a higher BV.

Some people who are on a low-fat or no-fat diet tend to be terrified of eating eggs or meats, for fear that these will make them fat or increase their cholesterol. I have been successfully lowering my patients' cholesterol readings for years, while allowing them to eat as many whole eggs as they wish. There are two important ingredients in an egg yolk, choline and inositol. These are great for improving fat metabolism and are also contained in a nutritional supplement that I sell to my patients to help them lower their cholesterol levels. Mother Nature knows how to design food!

BIOLOGIC VALUE OF DIETARY PROTEINS
Renner E. Milk Protein. In: *Milk and Dairy Products in Human Nutrition*,
Munich: Volkswirtschaftlicher Verlag; 1983

PROTEIN	BIOLOGIC VALUE(BV)
Lactalbumin (whey)	104
Egg	100
Cow's Milk	80
Beef	80
Fish	79
Casein (milk protein)	77
Soy	74
Potato	71
Rice	59
Wheat	54
Beans	49

The egg used to hold the place of honor at the top of this list; however, whey protein, which is the main constituent of mother's milk, is the very best protein. The proteins of cow's milk are composed of eighty percent casein and twenty percent whey protein. Casein has a much lower BV. Human milk has the opposite ratio, containing seventy to eighty percent whey protein.

This is the main reason babies are short-changed when being fed formulas derived from cow's milk, soy or rice proteins. The casein and lactose (milk sugar) in cow's milk are also a frequent source of allergy in infants. This allergy can cause excessive mucus and inflammation that contributes to upper respiratory infections and earaches. Please commit to breast-feeding your child for at least one year. It will have life-long benefits.

There are many medical uses of a high quality whey protein concentrate (WPC). These contain at least eighty percent protein with naturally occurring constituents, largely undenatured (not damaged), active and verified (both quantities and activity) by laboratory analysis. It is produced through an ultrafiltration/diafiltration, low heat, pH controlled process.

WPC contains all essential and non-essential amino acids. It is ideally suited to improve body composition (body fat ratio). WPC is high in cysteine and glutamine, two amino acids required to make glutathione. Glutathione is a key free-radical scavenger in the body, which is important in the prevention of cancer. Glutamine is also the predominant amino acid in skeletal muscle. It provides fuel and promotes growth to the rapidly dividing cells of the intestinal lining. It is also an important fuel for white blood cells and macrophages.

Another important immune benefit of WPC is that it contains protein molecules (immunoglobulins) that function as antibiodies against many harmful bacteria and viruses. Animal studies have shown that WPC was found to be as effective as colostrum in protecting newborn calves from disease. Furthermore, a lower level of the concentrated whey was required to provide this protection (twenty-seven grams of concentrated whey versus one hundred grams of colostrum).

Colostrum products are available through a number of sources but they are both expensive and occasionally unstable. **Metagenics** has developed a whey protein concentrate containing active immunoglobulins to promote the activity level of the immune system, nourish the intestinal tract and help gain lean muscle mass. It is called **BioPure Protein™**, and is available in a three hundred gram container.

THE BENEFITS OF SOY

As you can see from the Biologic Value chart, soy is head and shoulders above most beans when it comes to the quality of protein. This is why soy is a very popular additive to foods and protein drinks. In October of 1999, the U.S. **Food and Drug Administration** announced there was significant evidence of the benefit of eating twenty-five grams of soy protein daily. This quantity is said to lower cholesterol and the risk of coronary heart disease.

In addition, other studies are finding soy to be beneficial in reducing hot flashes, and lowering the risk of breast and prostate cancers. It may also prevent calcium loss and ward off osteoporosis. Perhaps this is one explanation for why Asians have less incidence of osteoporosis than Americans, despite the near non-existence of milk products in their diets.

Soy has a broad spectrum of isoflavones that seem to be responsible for its most beneficial anti-cancer and anti-cholesterol effects. **Archers Daniel Midland** manufactures a patented soy concentrate called **NovaSoy™**, which supplies a full spectrum of isoflavones, including genistein, diadzein, and glycitein. This product is found in a variety of soy products available in stores. **Metagenics** uses **NovaSoy™** in a product called **SpectraSoy®**, which provides forty-five milligrams of isoflavones per tablet.

Metagenics also provides seventeen mg. of soy isoflavones in a flavored protein beverage called **UltraMeal®**. This can be used as a meal substitute for weight management or snacks. I frequently recommend this to my clients who desire breakfast foods that do not contain wheat. **Ultrameal®** comes in four flavors and is easy to prepare, using two scoops mixed with water. It has an excellent booklet that describes a medically tested weight loss program combined with exercise that helps decrease body fat and increase lean muscle mass.

Another protein product by **Metagenics**, that is wonderful for breakfast, is their medical food specifically fortified for blood sugar regulation called **UltraGlycemX™**. This product also has seventeen mg. of soy isoflavones per serving. Both of the above products come with free color booklets (over thirty pages) that explain more about making better dietary choices, meal planning and several recipes.

Tofu is another great way to get your daily soy. I sometimes cook it for breakfast. Since it is rather bland, my favorite way to cook it is to just dip it in soy sauce briefly and fry both sides in a dry pan. You can also add this to stir-fry meals. It really is quite tasty!

Snacks

It is wise to choose foods with a higher protein content for your snacks so you can defend yourself against the mid-day slump. Skip the candy and pop machines and buy yourself a variety of nuts such as walnuts, almonds, pecans, and seeds like pumpkin and sunflower seeds. Buy all of these raw and in their whole form to prevent rancidity, and store them in the refrigerator.

I prefer the taste of dry roasting my nuts and seeds. I only do as many as I can consume in a week. To dry roast them, place them on a cookie sheet in a low-heat oven or put them in a dry skillet on medium-low heat on the stove. To prevent burning, mix them around to flip them over. Raw pumpkin seeds will start popping and jumping when heated, so keep an eye on them and turn the heat down.

Today's Activity

Now that your are more conscious of what foods contain protein, take a look back at your diet chart and see how much protein you have been consuming. Circle the protein foods and calculate whether you are getting at least sixty grams of protein per day.

"We make the world we live in
and shape our own environment."
— Orison Swett Marden

3 Day Food & Activity Diary

	Date:	Date:	Date:
Morning Meal Time:			
Snack			
Noon Meal Time:			
Snack			
Evening Meal Time:			
Snack			
Symptoms (Physical & Emotional)			
Exercise Type & Duration			

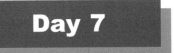

Day 7

"We more frequently fail to face the right problem
than fail to solve the problem we face."

—Unknown

Simple Methods of Mineral Deficiency Analysis

Mineral deficiency is extremely common among Americans due to the depletion of minerals in our agricultural soils and the excessive consumption of refined foods which utilize several minerals in their metabolism. Toxic minerals, such as the heavy metals: lead, mercury, arsenic, cadmium, aluminum etc. are another significant problem contributing to deficiency of our nutritional minerals. They displace many of our important minerals such as calcium. We ingest heavy metals in water, breathe them in the air (and from cigarette smoke), get exposed to them in our workplace and even receive them in conjunction with medicines and dental work.

A review by the **Food and Drug Administration** in July, 1999 indicated that pediatricians are starting to get concerned by the number of vaccinations using a mercury preservative. They are beginning to study whether the increasing number of required vaccinations might be pushing infants over the toxicity guidelines.

The **National Research Council** has also cautioned that more than sixty thousand American children a year are born at risk of nerve or brain damage from mercury exposure in the womb. Mercury is produced by incinerators and coal-burning power plants. The Great Lakes area has a significant problem with mercury-tainted fish. Fetuses are especially vulnerable when their mothers eat such fish because their brains are growing so fast. A coalition of seven consumer groups sent a letter to the director of the **U.S. Health and Human Services** in January, 2001 to request that the **FDA** warn pregnant and nursing mothers and young children to sharply decrease consumption of fish such as shark, swordfish, mackerel and tuna steaks. People who are at risk for mercury toxicity should be tested before they exhibit neurological symptoms. Signs of chronic mercury poisoning include unsteadiness, tremors, irritability, and depression.

Moderate levels of arsenic can cause abdominal pain, vomiting, diarrhea, and muscle cramps. Long-term exposure to lead can also cause abdominal pain, constipation, headaches, and irritability. Common sources of lead exposure include paints, pottery and candle wicks. Lead exposure in children has been linked to mental impairment and a decrease in IQ. **Dr. Herbert Needleman** of the **University of Pittsburgh** also found a strong link between lead exposure and juvenile delinquency. An example of how heavy metals can displace other minerals was noted in an article published in the **Journal of the American Medical Association** on June 23, 1999, which found an association between lead and tooth decay that may affect as many as 2.7 million children.

TESTING FOR MINERAL DEFICIENCY

When a new patient comes into my office, I do a simple test known as the *Zinc Tally Test* to determine if their bodies are deficient in zinc. This is the only mineral that can be easily tested in an office. If zinc is extremely low, it is important to test for other mineral deficiencies.

Since zinc deficiency decreases the sense of taste, we simply ask the patient to hold a small amount of liquid zinc in their mouth and then count how long it takes for them to taste a chalky or metallic flavor. The zinc test solution is called **Zinc Tally™**, and is available from **Metagenics.**

A person who is well nourished with zinc will immediately experience an obnoxious taste. For those who are deficient it will first taste like water. If they still do not taste it by about twenty seconds, their first awareness will usually just be a mild chalkiness. I have many patients who regularly take a multivitamin, and still cannot taste the zinc after fifty seconds. At this point I stop the test and just have them swallow the zinc. I then either supplement zinc with their multivitamin, until the *Zinc Tally Test* becomes normal or I assess their overall mineral status with a **Hair Elemental Analysis** by **Great Smokies Diagnostic Lab**, (see Resources).

People who often need extra zinc are those with frequent colds, sore throats, indigestion, slow healing of wounds and men with prostate problems. **Metagenics** provides zinc either in a tablet form, (**Zinc AG™**) or a liquid form, which is stronger than Zinc Tally, known as **Zinc Drink™**. The liquid form is useful for someone who would benefit from gargling with zinc – those with gum disease, sore throats or colds. **Metagenics** also makes Zinc lozenges (**ZincAid Plus™**) for support throughout the day for an infection.

AMAZING STORIES THE HAIR CAN TELL

Hair analysis is a very inexpensive and helpful way to assess your total mineral status. It provides a convenient method of gauging chronic toxic exposure and nutrient mineral deficiencies in the body. This test can help identify mineral imbalances that may be triggering problems such as chronic fatigue, depression, attention deficits, hyperactivity disorders, violent behavior, reactivity to stress, arthritis, cardiovascular disease, glucose intolerance, allergic stress and thyroid deficiency.

Hair analysis is a laboratory test that has been around a long time. Over the past eighteen years of my practice I have seen a variety of tests performed at different laboratories. The quality of testing we now have available far surpasses the accuracy we were able to obtain in the early days of my practice.

The accuracy and reliability of this test depends on the integrity of the sample, proper administration, and the technique of the laboratory. **Great Smokies Diagnostic Laboratory** has taken the technology to new heights. I am not aware of any other company that can display results that reflect the accuracy of a mineral value that pertains only to the patient's hair and warns of external contamination altering the readings.

The following are examples of the aformentioned hair analysis testing and technology available through **Great Smokies Laboratory**.

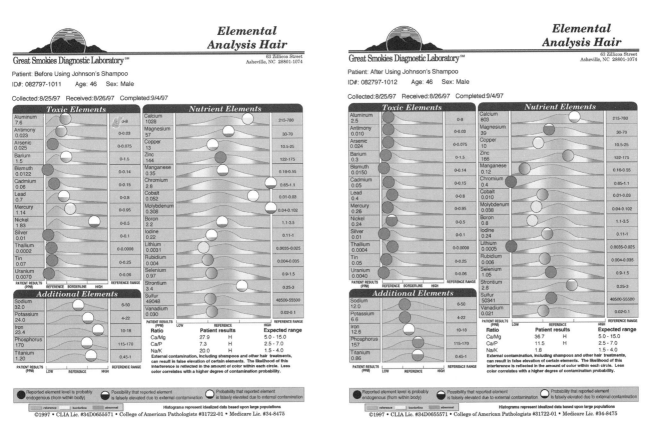

Figure 7.1

Figure 7.1 shows two samples from the same person with the results altered significantly just by preparing the hair properly with **Johnson and Johnson's** baby shampoo. Their test indicates the accuracy of the reading for each mineral by showing a solid circle for an accurate reading and then varying degrees of external contamination by a circle with a "water line" showing part solid and part white. The more white present, the more unreliable the result for that mineral. The shades of gray reflect whether the result is in the normal or abnormal range and do not relate to external contamination.

You can see that for most minerals, the results are not even close. Sometimes, even with using the shampoo there are other contaminants that cause inaccurate readings. Therefore, high or low values that **Great Smokies** deems to be inaccurate will not falsely lead the clinician to make improper recommendations. For more information on the controversy regarding reliability of hair mineral testing, visit **www.gsdl.com**.

GREAT SMOKIES DIAGNOSTIC LABORATORY FEELS THAT THE FOLLOWING PRE-TEST CRITERIA ARE CRUCIAL FOR AN ACCURATE SAMPLING:

- Use **Johnson and Johnson's "No More Tears"** shampoo for at least a week prior to the test.
- Avoid selenium (dandruff) shampoos for two months prior to the test – selenium does not wash out.
- Wait two months after hair has been dyed or permed to take a sample. Samples are typically taken from the back of the head and sometimes you can avoid chemical treatments to that area.
- Do not take specimens within two months of general anesthesia. This causes hair to stop growing and increases the concentration of almost all hair elements as much as two to three times normal.
- Avoid chlorinated pools and mineral baths for two weeks prior to collection. Well water and copper plumbing can also be a source of contamination.
- Avoid conditioners, mousse or other preparations the day of the hair collection. Make sure the hair is completely dry.
- Cut the hair with stainless steel scissors wiped with a cloth dampened with water. Do not shave the hair or use electric clippers.
- For those with baldness, pubic hair can be utilized. However, it commonly has greater levels of aluminum, nickel, sodium, potassium and phosphorus and much less sulfur than scalp hair.

HAIR ANALYSIS FOR FATIGUE

The hair analysis can offer valuable information to someone with fatigue. It will identify whether your body is overburdened by toxic elements. Elevation of cadmium, lead, silver and mercury can come from the ingestion of shellfish. Mercury elevation can be related to the ingestion of large ocean fish or fish from any body of water polluted by "acid rain."

Mercury from old dental amalgam fillings will not show up on the hair mineral analysis. This is best tested with the **Great Smokies'** urine mineral analysis. Sometimes an oral chelating agent is administered for a few days prior to testing.

Smoking can cause elevated lead, cadmium, nickel, silver and tin, with higher levels of lead and cadmium seen in those who smoke marijuana. Many of these minerals will also be present in the hair of those exposed to second-hand smoke. Antacids, deodorant, cooking pots and foil can be a cause for elevated aluminum. Colloidal mineral supplements can also cause an elevated aluminum. These products are derived from the earth's crust, where alluminum is the most plentiful mineral present.

The hair mineral analysis can also identify malabsorption of minerals: sometimes from insufficient stomach acid or the frequent use of antacids or acid blockers. Deficient stomach acid is often seen with low levels of zinc and chromium. Symptoms of zinc deficiency are a decreased sense of taste and smell, which causes cravings for salty and spicy food. Zinc-deficient individuals also tend to experience more bloating and gas after meals.

Low levels of calcium, magnesium and zinc can not only show up as abnormally low but also as abnormally high. This is due to abnormal deposition in the hair and other tissues from prolonged deficiency of these elements. This makes them unavailable to the tissues that need them. Magnesium is one of the most important minerals for energy production. Depressed magnesium has also been associated with depression, increased cardiac risk and hypertension.

Low levels of iodine can be the first sign of low thyroid function, a cause of both fatigue and depression. Low lithium levels can also suggest risk of depression, especially when combined with low magnesium. Low levels of the minerals chromium and/or vanadium can indicate hypoglycemia or diabetes. Low chromium can also be a factor in weight problems, both underweight and excessive weight. Low cobalt can indicate vitamin B12 deficiency, a common form of anemia.

Allergies or B6 deficiency can show up with depressed levels of calcium, magnesium, manganese, chromium and cobalt. Sodium, potassium and zinc are usually elevated with these conditions.

MINERAL DEFICIENCY AND BEHAVIOR DISORDERS

Because attention deficit disorder and hyperactivity are treated with stimulant drugs, which can ultimately exhaust the body, I want to end this chapter with a discussion of what hair analysis can offer to behavior disorders. There are categories of behavior disorders defined by **Dr. Bill Walsh** of the **Pfeiffer Treatment Center** of Naperville, IL. He has found patterns of abnormal hair element levels in many subjects affected by these disorders.

1) **Type A behavior** is common in children with behavior disorders and in many aggressive adults. Common characteristics include attention deficit disorders, under-achievement, susceptibility to sunburn, allergies, remorse after wrong-doing, frequent violence, and a Jekyll-Hyde behavior pattern among males.

Hair analysis patterns, in Type A behavior, include depressed or elevated calcium and magnesium, depressed sodium and potassium, elevated levels of one or more toxic elements, elevated manganese, and deficiency of zinc, chromium, cobalt and lithium.

Elevated manganese has been seen in children with learning problems and in many perpetrators of domestic violence. Manganese has been commonly used as a gasoline additive since they removed lead from gas. Perhaps this may relate to the increase in road rage along congested highways.

2) **Type B behavior** is present in extremely violent individuals. Typical characteristics of these individuals include sleeplessness, a high threshold for pain, frequent aggressive behavior, an absence of remorse, obsessive-compulsive behavior, high sexual drive, a fascination with fire and pathological lying. Type B patients will often respond quickly to supplementation, showing improvement in as little as a week.

The hair analysis of Type B's typically shows elevation of multiple toxic elements. Zinc is the nutrient element most often deviated (high or low). Lithium and cobalt are commonly depressed, a situation that has been associated with the degree of violence. The lower the levels, the more likely the violence. Additionally, many of the elements sensitive to vitamin B6 levels are depressed.

3) **Type C behavior** pattern relates to people who are delinquent, mildly aggressive, underachievers, argumentative and impulsive. They do not usually hurt others. Often they have malabsorption and digestive problems.

Their hair usually shows decreased levels of calcium, magnesium and zinc, which can also appear as abnormally high. Type C behavior usually exhibits low copper and manganese. Their blood plasma frequently shows low levels of amino acids.

4) **Type D behavior** pattern is seen much more in males than females. This type commonly exhibits mild aggressive tendencies, is often comprised of delinquent individuals and underachievers, may be argumentative, slender, and impulsive. These individuals sometimes commit petty thefts and seldom maintain a driver's license. They often have malabsorption problems and are usually low in plasma amino acids.

Their hair often shows multiple low minerals such as chromium, manganese, calcium, magnesium and zinc. Copper, cobalt, molybdenum and vanadium are also often depressed due to insufficient stomach acid.

Information for this chapter has been collected from the **Elemental Analysis Hair Interpretive Guidelines** available for licensed professional healthcare providers by **Great Smokies Diagnostic Laboratory,** Asheville, N.C., **www.gsdl.com**

> "The real contest is always between what you've done and what you're capable of doing. You measure yourself against yourself and nobody else."
> — Geoffry Gaberino

Day 8

Love & Forgive

Maintaining good health requires that you make important choices every day, regarding not only your body, but also your mind and spirit. Our thoughts can powerfully create our reality. If we are tired or sick we need to examine our thoughts to determine whether we are thinking **constructively** or **destructively**. With that in mind, please consider the following "Love Resolutions:"

Love Resolution #1: **Resolve to give up, for one month (and hopefully longer!), one food, beverage or activity that is an unhealthy habit or addiction.**

When we give up our time, money, health and power to excessive or unhealthy habits, we are being disrespectful to our physical and emotional well-being. These behaviors are not only detrimental to our health, but may interfere with our personal relationships and even our occupations.

Many behavioral experts agree it takes twenty-one days of consistent effort to break an old habit. The chart on page sixty-one will assist you in developing a course of action for breaking unhealthy habits. You will be surprised how easy some of these habits are to break. Many of these items are not ones you have to give up entirely. Someone who is a food binger certainly cannot stop eating! The foods and beverages I listed are either energy depleters or common food allergens and **should not be consumed daily.**

Once you have broken the addiction cycle on foods such as flour, sugar, or dairy products, you will be able to occasionally return to them without losing control. Some of the old **daily** habits can now become something you can enjoy once a week or once a month without backsliding. If they start **controlling you** again, stick with abstinence until your body becomes better nourished.

One of the latest trends in the treatment of alcoholism is to help the person discontinue habits of daily alcohol consumption or binging by allowing them to drink in moderation on special occasions. For some people, this is more successful than total abstinence, which has been the hallmark of **Alcoholics Anonymous** for over sixty years. If a person is well nourished and controlling their hypoglycemia and insulin imbalances, they will be less likely to binge on foods or alcohol.

An excellent book on the relationship of alcoholism to hypoglycemia and nutritional imbalances is **Seven Weeks to Sobriety** by **Joan Mathews Larson, Ph.D**. She is the director of the alcoholism treatment facility,

Health Recovery Center, in Minneapolis. This program has a seventy-five percent success rate, three times higher than conventional treatment programs, because it focuses on correcting nutrient depletions caused by alcoholism.

Consider tackling as many of the problems in the first list as you can. Prominent Functional Medicine practitioner, **Sidney Baker, M.D.**, describes the "Tacks Rule" when trying to improve chronic health problems. It goes something like this: "Imagine sitting in a chair with ten tacks. If you remove only three of them, will it feel much better?"

Do not berate yourself for backsliding on any of these goals. Focus on getting back to what you desire to change. The past is a closed chapter. The present and future are yet to be written and are filled with exciting choices. You have the ability to make more powerful choices and realize your full potential. Claim your power over these habits and stop wasting energy that can be used to achieve greater goals.

> "First we form habits, then they form us.
> Conquer your bad habits or they will conquer you."
> —Rob Gilbert

Observe what benefits and problems come up during this time. Note what you substitute for the habit. Is it a healthier choice? Does total abstinence make it easier or more difficult? Examine how it affects your relationships. Is anyone trying to sabotage your success? This is *extremely* common. Do your friends get mad at you for being a "party pooper?" Or do you have more time for face-to-face relationships because you are not wasting all of your free time in front of the TV or computer?

I have noticed at banquets or parties how some people feel uncomfortable eating desserts, etc. in front of me. They assume I will frown on their indulgence. People who know me better understand that my message is not a "guilt-trip" of never-never. I stress that healthy people should make the best choices for their health ninety percent of the time and then enjoy the party. People with chronic illness may have to be more vigilant about avoiding depleted foods. Most people are making poor health choices far too often.

Spend some time thinking of a wonderful reward for your efforts. Use the money, previously spent on the addiction, for something you have needed and have put off buying for a long time. Go dancing or take a yoga class with the extra time you have. Write letters or catch up on a former hobby you have put aside.

This is also a good time to clean out some clutter and either hold a big garage sale or donate your cast-offs. Nothing signals to the world that you are ready for a change more than throwing out things you no longer want in your life. It creates an opening for greater things to come.

TODAY'S ACTIVITY

BREAKING COMMON HABITS AND ADDICTIONS

1. Consider the following list of common habits or addictions. The first group is foods and beverages. The second group is activities, tobacco and drugs.

2. Check off that apply to you. Be sure to write down your present activity in *all* these areas even if you presently have no plans to alter these habits.

3. Circle the ones you would like to work on this month.

4. Decide whether you want to work on total abstinence or just a significant decrease in activity and state that goal. There are exactly twenty-one days left before you reach "Graduation Day." Good luck!

5. Return to this list at the end of the thirty-day wellness program to see which ones you have successfully changed. At that time, write goals for three months for *each* of the items you originally checked. There may be some you are still not ready to tackle. Change takes time. Congratulate yourself for moving in the right direction!

Common Habit/Addiction	Present Activity	21 Day Goal	Progress at End of Program	3 Month Goal
Ex. √ soda	*2 cans/day*	*1/week*	*1/month*	*rarely*
☐ soda				
☐ caffeine				
☐ chocolate				
☐ sugar				
☐ donuts/pastry				
☐ candy				
☐ alcohol				
☐ dairy				
☐ snack foods				

Common Habit/Addiction	Present Activity	21 Day Goal	Progress at End of Program	3 Month Goal
Ex.: √ cigarettes	*2 packs/day*	*10/day*	*1 pack/week*	*quit*
☐ tobacco				
☐ illegal drugs				
☐ television				
☐ computer games				
☐ gambling/lotto				
☐ pornography				
☐ other:				

Love Resolution #2: Resolve to forgive someone who has wronged you.

This is not a sign of weakness but a sign of strength; to be able to stop wasting energy on negative thoughts that are harming you. As long as you are spending time on disturbing thoughts from the past, you are diminishing your ability to put energy into new and exciting endeavors and relationships. Put an end to the bitterness!

Forgiving someone does not mean you condone their behavior or are letting them "off the hook." It means you are taking *yourself* off the hook, which you have been dangling from. Imagine your feet hanging a foot off the ground, unable to move forward, backward or sideways. This is the mental trap you create when you refuse to forgive and let go.

Do not allow yourself to let this issue continue to hold back your life. Break through to a higher level of functioning. Forgiveness is your ticket to freedom. It will bring you tremendous blessings.

TODAY'S ACTIVITY

FORGIVENESS

Who is one person you would like to forgive? _____

How would *you* benefit if you forgave this person?_____

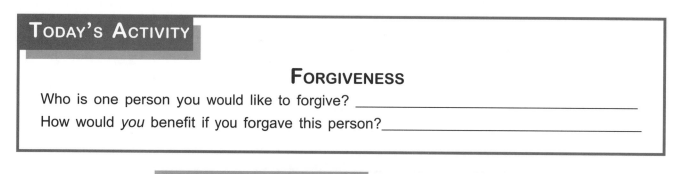

"Man must evolve for all human conflict, a method which rejects revenge, aggression and retaliation. The foundation of such a method is love."
— Dr. Martin Luther King Jr.

Love Resolution #3: Resolve to stop living a lie.

I once read that a major cause of depression was dishonesty. Since most depressed people report being fatigued, we need to explore this issue. Cheating on your spouse, misrepresenting yourself or being dishonest in your business dealings are very stressful to your health.

The energy you spend covering up a lie drains an exponential amount of energy from your life. Even suppressing anger and outwardly appearing sweet and agreeable can take a huge toll on your health. This is a common pattern of behavior among arthritis sufferers. They suppress their anger because someone once told them it was not okay to get mad.

PERSONAL STORY

My parents are a prime example of how a huge lie poisoned their entire marriage. Before their wedding my mother became pregnant. My father (who was raised Catholic) would not marry her in her pregnant condition so he forced her to get an abortion – 1940's style. My mother never forgave herself for yielding to his wishes and it killed the love she once felt for him. She was also angered by my father's dishonest practice of his religion and would have nothing to do with Catholicism. She had various health problems the rest of her life. When their fiftieth wedding anniversary came around she viewed it as one of the biggest failures of her life and refused to celebrate the occasion. She died two months later.

Never underestimate the power of confession to heal dishonesty. Keeping a dark secret can create spiritual and emotional conflict for an entire family. My mother confessed her abortion to us long before she died and it helped my sisters and me understand the discord between them. Before my father died I asked him to discuss this issue with his priest and I am very thankful he did. Until that time, I do not believe he realized how much it had emotionally impacted him for over fifty years.

Trying to run from misdeeds in your past will never lead to freedom. If you do, you will never enjoy your future. Prayer, confession and forgiveness are all important elements to resolve past conflicts.

TODAY'S ACTIVITY

BEING HONEST

Write down an example of dishonesty in your life that you wish to change:

_____

HELPFUL TOOLS

One of the first books to examine the correlation between thoughts, disease and the body parts afflicted is **Louise Hay's** timeless booklet titled, ***Heal Your Body,*** written in 1982. Almost the entire booklet is a chart of various health conditions with headings such as, "The Problem," "Probable Cause," and "New Thought Pattern." It contains affirmations to use in meditation to help you work through the conflict.

Another book, which explores more deeply how the parts of the body become entangled with the psyche and create disease, is **Serge King's, *Imagineering For Health***. An interesting idea I gained from this book is his explanation of how the chest is our "Identity Center." When we point to ourselves and say "Me," we do not point to our head or our waist. We point to our chest.

King states, "The chest is where our body harbors ideas relating to self-worth, rejection, compassion, assertiveness, pride or humility." It is probably a factor in why women who have a weak sense of identity or low level of self-confidence feel compelled to have breast augmentation. Breast and lung cancers often come about after your identity changes, for instance, after the loss of a spouse or change in occupation or retirement.

PHYSICAL/EMOTIONAL RELATIONSHIPS

Oriental Medicine has long recognized the relationship of the body and emotions. From their perspective, denying your feelings, hiding your true emotions from others, or excessive expression of certain emotions can all cause you to become ill. A predominant emotion can also be the first sign of an organ suffering dysfunction. For instance, the liver and gall bladder are associated with anger and shouting. Excessive anger or hostility can be one of the earliest warning signs that the liver is overburdened by such things as alcohol, caffeine, drugs or increased toxic exposure from our environment. Many drugs, including over the counter pain relievers, have warning labels regarding liver toxicity.

The heart and small intestine are associated with both joy and anxiety, laughing and being talkative. Anyone who suffers from panic attacks can attest to the frightening symptoms associated with the heart. The spleen and pancreas are associated with worry, obsession, indecision and suspicion.

The lungs and large intestine are associated with grief, sadness and depression. If someone has a death in the family they are more prone to pneumonia, bronchitis, or colitis afterward. The kidneys and bladder are associated with fear and insecurity. When you consider our adrenals sit right on top of our kidneys, you can understand how the "fight or flight" reaction to fearful events can influence these organs. People with chronically stressed adrenals often suffer from frequent urination.

Love Resolution #4:   Resolve to stop hating your body.

Hatred toward your body's fat, attractiveness, flexibility, strength, endurance or an unpleasant symptom will never change any of those things for the better. Shame and hatred are both choices. You *can* consciously decide to stop giving these emotions power over your life. Recognize how much valuable time you have wasted on that kind of negative energy and resolve to drop those attitudes.

When a disease disables or disfigures you, it is very common to go through emotions that are similar to those experienced within a person who is dying – grief, anger, and acceptance. In reality, it is the death of your old self you are grieving for and mad about losing. The healing comes when you can truly accept your appearance and state of health and truly prosper from the experience.

PERSONAL STORY

Over the twenty years of my autoimmune illness, I wasted far too many days being angry toward my body, mad at God, and envious of everyone else who was not afflicted. One day at work I was absolutely wallowing in a "pity party" of shame, disgust and hatred about how the skin on my arms and legs had been damaged from the severe itching of my disease. I had a free hour before a new patient was to arrive so I was really doing a number on myself. At the appointed time the patient arrived and luckily, she turned out to be an angel from God.

"Janelle" was about my age and had been burned about five years previously over seventy percent of her body, including her face. She had already endured over thirty operations and was scheduled to have many more. I was so ashamed of myself I almost burst into tears right in front of her. This woman became my friend and I will always love her for the lessons she has taught me about self-love and acceptance. She is now happily married and working again.

Accept what cannot be changed and take action steps toward improving what can be changed. Resolve to spend ten minutes per day on an activity that enhances the way you feel about yourself -- even if it is just staring at yourself in the mirror and saying, "I love and accept you" to yourself.

That simple activity helped one woman, **Evy McDonald**, become the first documented case of recovery from the fatal and crippling disease, ALS or Lou Gehrig's disease. In 1980, Evy was given one year to live, at most. She decided in her last months of life she wanted to experience unconditional love. She realized she had always hated her body so she devised a way to make a radical change.

Evy sat naked in her wheelchair in front of a mirror and committed herself to find a least one new thing every day to love about herself. Over time, her ALS mysteriously reversed its couse and her body experienced an unprecedented recovery. I heard of Evy from singer and songwriter, **Greg Tamblyn**, who has written a beautiful song about her entitled, "**Unconditional Love (The Story of Evy)**." It is found on his CD, "**The Shootout at the I'm OK, You're OK Corral**," ® 1992, **Tunetown Records**, P.O. Box 45258, Kansas City, Missouri 64171, **www.gregtamblyn.com**.

> "Love is the immortal flow of energy that nourishes, extends and preserves. Its eternal goal is life."
> —Smiley Blanton

TODAY'S ACTIVITY

SELF-LOVE

What do you most love about yourself or your body? _____

Take something you presently dislike about yourself and turn it into a statement that will convince your subconscious mind that you love it just as much as what you wrote above. For instance, "I have abundant energy and vitality!" _____

_____

Love Resolution #5:   Resolve to send out mental messages of love daily.

Send out mental messages of love to people you meet, your loved ones near and far, and countries that are struggling with war or poverty. Unfortunately, it is so much easier to view others unlike ourselves with suspicion and even hatred. "Guilty until proven innocent," seems to be the attitude many people take.

PERSONAL STORY

Over the years I have come to understand that those who spread a blanket of hatred over entire races or groups are actually retaliating against a former abuse or enduring a very deep self-hatred they are afraid to face.

In junior high school I became a bully against a very shy and quiet girl, whom I taunted with verbal insults. It was fifteen years later that I recognized I was trying to overcome feelings of being powerless against a person close to me who was physically and emotionally abusing me. I was looking for someone weak, whom I could overpower, to prove I was really strong after all. In reality, I was developing a persona among my peers of being nasty, uncompassionate and of weak character.

When I got to high school I added a mildly retarded girl to my list. Thankfully, soon afterward a senior girl yelled at me to stop. It made me realize how obnoxious and unkind my behavior had been. Thankfully, I did not waste any more years being so unloving toward others. It is impossible to project hatred toward others without causing harm to your own body and soul.

This incident also points out the importance of intervention when you see acts that are unjust. So often we are afraid of getting involved. That senior not only protected the girls I was abusing, she made me a better person. It reminds me of the WWJD movement which stands for "What Would Jesus Do?" That young woman definitely acted like Jesus in that situation and helped bring healing to all involved.

SMILE!

The power of a simple smile was made strikingly evident to me one day at a seminar. The presenter asked an audience member to participate and proceeded to do a muscle strength test with the arm out laterally ninety degrees. Then he quickly drew a smiley face and asked the person to look at the picture while he muscle tested again. The muscle had been strong both times. Next, he quickly drew a similar picture with a frown, held it up in front of his subject and muscle tested again. This time the person's arm went weak. I have repeated this test several times with similar results.

Try this test with your friends. It will burn an impression on your heart about the importance of sending love and positive energy to your loved ones with a simple smile. When was the last time you smiled at your spouse or your children? Notice the difference between how you look at those people you like and those you do not. The only difference may be whether they smile at you. Smile at them and break the ice! Perhaps the only thing between you and this person becoming great friends is a sour expression.

Become aware of how easily children smile at others and how some adults never seem to smile. Recent research found that children laugh about four hundred times per day! Think of how much more pleasant our world would be if we greeted each other with a smile!

The power of our expression and tone of voice became very evident to me when my son was an infant. Like any parent, I lost my temper a few times and shouted at him. All three times my son developed a fever that evening which was gone by morning. I learned a valuable lesson about the destructive power of angry words.

TODAY'S ACTIVITY

SMILE!

Twenty four hours from now write down how many people you made an extra effort to smile at: _____

THE POWER OF PRAYER

The power of prayer is receiving much attention as a method to heal others, even when people do not know they are being prayed for. One of my favorite stories about the amazing power of healing prayer is contained in the first edition of *Chicken Soup For the Soul*, by **Mark Victor Hansen** and **Jack Canfield.**

It involved a young woman named **Amy Graham** who was predicted to die of leukemia in less than a week. Her parents contacted the **Make A Wish Foundation** and said that Amy's last wish was to meet Mark Victor Hansen and attend his seminar. Mark was absolutely astonished this child would value experiencing his seminar as her dying wish.

At the end of his seminar he felt compelled to tell his audience the story of this young woman and asked her to come up on the stage. At this point she was too weak to walk without the assistance of her father. He asked his audience if they would rub their hands together to build up heat and then extend their hands and send healing energy to Amy. Two weeks later she called Mark to report that she was in total remission. Two years later she contacted him with the great news that she was about to be married.

The best part is that this was not just an isolated incident. I have heard of many spontaneous healings through the power of prayer. They are happening both in religious and secular circles. What a miraculous gift from our Creator!

> "Too often we underestimate the power of a touch,
> a smile, a kind word, a listening ear,
> an honest compliment, or the smallest act of caring,
> all of which have the potential to turn a life around."
> -- Leo Buscaglia

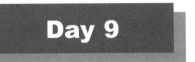

Take a Breathing Break

I have a theory about smoking. I believe the reason smokers consider this a calming and relaxing habit is because they are actually doing a five-minute breathing exercise. Think about it — if instead of smoking we took a five-minute break several times a day to concentrate on deep breathing, we would become much more energized and relaxed. Since there are twenty cigarettes in a pack, those with a two-pack-a-day habit are taking *forty breathing breaks per day!* WOW! What are we nonsmokers missing out on?

Consider oxygen to be one of your most important nutrients. When we are under chronic stress we automatically go into a pattern of very shallow breathing. Your whole posture can sometimes look like your chest is collapsed. When you are not breathing well, your entire body feels low on energy. Everyone feels better after taking a walk in the fresh air.

There was a study done in the 1990's that measured the carbon monoxide content in the blood of a jogger who was running along a very smoggy highway in Los Angeles. They compared it to the blood of a person of similar age and size who was driving a car along the same highway with the windows rolled up and the air conditioner on. You guessed it. The jogger was detoxifying the carbon monoxide from his body better than the driver!

I would like to start a national craze of "Breathing Breaks!" There are three very simple breathing techniques you can do almost anywhere. You can focus on these when you are walking, working, driving a car, watching TV or participating in a tense business meeting. Of course, these techniques would be most effective if you could do them when you are able to focus entirely on your breathing.

For more information on breathing techniques and their benefits, I can recommend an excellent CD recorded by **Dr. Andrew Weil**, who is a well-known author and Director of the Program in Integrative Medicine at the **University of Arizona** in Tucson. It is called *Breathing – The Master Key to Self Healing* and is available in major bookstores that offer CD's.

Dr. Weil reports that these breathing exercises bring him more favorable responses from patients than anything else he teaches. He explains how proper breathing has the remarkable ability to reprogram the nervous system to achieve benefits such as increasing energy, lowering blood pressure, improving circulation and overcoming anxiety disorders.

TODAY'S ACTIVITY

BREATHING EXERCISES

Breathing Exercise #1: The first method involves exhaling twice as long as you inhale. Imagine this to be a detoxifying exercise because exhaling is a great way for your body to rid itself of toxic gases. Set your watch or a kitchen timer for five minutes. Sit in a comfortable chair and make sure your breastbone is lifted instead of collapsed into your chest. Put your hand on your abdomen to make sure your belly expands when you inhale.

Unless your nose is very congested, try to breathe with your mouth closed. Inhale to the count of two and exhale to the count of four. If that feels like too short of a breathing interval go to three and six seconds of inhale/exhale. Some of you may prefer to do four and eight or five and ten. Now isn't this an amazing alternative to cigarettes! Can you imagine how you would feel if you remembered to do that twenty to forty times per day? No wonder smokers have difficulty quitting!

Breathing Exercise #2: This technique is similar to the previous one, but involves equal time for both the inhalation and exhalation. Note whether you can increase the number of seconds you can inhale after awhile.

The best part of these first two techniques is that no one has to know you are in the middle of taking a "Breathing Break." You can do them during all those boring moments in life, such as standing in line at the grocery store or while waiting for your computer to download information.

Breathing Exercise #3: This exercise helps to balance out the right and left sides of the brain, and helps to normalize imbalances in the activity between the Sympathetic and Parasympathetic nervous systems. Our Sympathetic nervous system is known as our "fight or flight" response mechanism, which is our way of reacting to danger. Unfortunately, many people have the Sympathetic nervous system in overdrive from being over-stimulated by caffeine, ephedrine, excessive work and meeting deadlines, video games, violent movies, etc.

The Parasympathetic nervous system is affectionately called the "rest and digest" part of the nervous system. This correctly implies that you will digest your food better if you are in a restful and calm mood. This is another reason why fast food and driving do not mix!

This breathing exercise is also known as "Alternate Breathing" because you will alternately breathe in one nostril and out the other. You can do this by covering nostrils with the thumb and index finger of one hand. This technique is a little harder to disguise while out in public. The best time to do this is before a meal or at bedtime because it is so beneficial for quieting your mind.

Activity continued on next page...

TODAY'S ACTIVITY CONTINUED

1.   First take a big breath with your mouth closed.
2.   Cover one nostril with your thumb and exhale air out of the remaining nostril.
3.   Inhale through the same nostril and then cover up both nostrils for a few seconds.
4.   Open the nostril you first covered with your thumb and exhale.
5.   Inhale through the same nostril and then close both nostrils.
6.   Repeat this sequence for about five minutes. You will always have one nostril that seems more open and this will change at times during the same day.

Remember to do your breathing exercises often throughout the day. Use mental triggers to remind you, such as seeing someone smoking, stopping at a red light, or hearing the heat or air conditioner turn on.

SMOKING

I have taught these techniques to many clients over the years who wanted to quit smoking. Many have told me it became effortless to gradually decrease their habit. Doing one of these techniques prior to lighting up often makes people desire to smoke only a few puffs of the cigarette.

Researchers have found that nicotine addiction is sometimes more difficult to break than addiction to illegal drugs. The previous chapter discussed overcoming several types of addictions. In my practice, I do not ask my clients to tackle smoking addiction first. It has been my experience that you will be more successful after you adopt dietary and lifestyle changes.

Overcoming tobacco and illegal drug addictions will be easier when your health is stronger. Use the breathing techniques to decrease your tobacco use over the next three weeks. At the end of this program, you will have a greater sense of personal power and will be much more ready to take on the bigger challenge of quitting altogether.

If you want further motivation to quit smoking, consider a study published in the ***British Medical Journal*** on August 3, 2000, which stated that giving up smoking even late in life eliminates the majority of risk for lung cancer. There is a ninety percent decrease in the risk for lung cancer in those who quit before they turned thirty-five. In Great Britain the number of lung cancer deaths has decreased by one-half since they started widely dropping the smoking habit around 1950.

Smoking has more immediate dangers than lung cancer. It can contribute to cardiovascular problems such as heart attacks, strokes and hypertension. It can also cause gum disease. Most recently, it has been discovered as a risk factor in colon cancer.

A study published in the March 9, 2000, ***New England Journal of Medicine***, found smokers were over four times more likely to get life-threatening blood infections or meningitis from a type of bacteria that usually causes pneumonia. This research was compiled by the **Centers for Disease Control** in Atlanta, Baltimore and Toronto and involved the organism, ***Streptococcus pneumoniae***. They found that those who smoked at least twenty-five cigarettes per day were five and one half times more likely to contract these infections. This news should be disturbing to college students, who are more commonly affected by meningitis outbreaks.

COLLEGE SMOKERS

Many college students in the U.S. are not paying heed to the anti-tobacco message. A 1999 **Harvard College Alcohol Survey** of more than fourteen thousand students found that:

- 45.7% said they had used tobacco within the past year
- 32.9 % said they had used a tobacco product within the past month
- 23% had smoked a cigar within the past year
- 8.5% had smoked a cigar within the past month

It was encouraging to note the novelty of smoking seemed to have worn off by the time students had graduated--more freshmen and sophomores used tobacco than juniors and seniors.

SMOKING AND PREGNANCY

There are big health concerns for pregnant women who smoke. Smoking can result in low birth weight, increased risk of stillbirth and learning and behavioral problems in children.

A study of over four thousand males, born in Denmark, between 1958 and 1961, found those born to pregnant women who smoked run a risk of violent and criminal behavior that lasts well into adulthood. The researchers believed this was caused by damage to the fetuses' central nervous systems. This study was published in the March, 1999 issue of the ***Archives of General Psychiatry.***

Another study done by **Steven Hecht**, of the **University of Minnesota Cancer Center,** found the presence of a smoking-related carcinogen, called NNK, in the urine of babies immediately after birth. The study suggested the need for more research to determine if the exposure of a carcinogen to a fetus throughout its gestation may increase the risk of childhood cancers.

In 1996, twelve percent of pregnant women admitted to smoking, with an average of fifteen cigarettes per day. But there is evidence that pregnant women are not always honest about their use of tobacco and drugs. A study of 970 women, who sought emergency treatment for miscarriage, at the **Hospital of the University of Pennsylvania** in Philadelphia, was reported in the February 4, 1999 issue of the ***New England Journal of Medicine.***

They used hair and urine tests to determine if a woman's reporting of the use of smoking and cocaine was reliable. They found that thirty-five percent of the women who miscarried were smokers, while only thirty percent admitted smoking cigarettes. Smokers were almost twice as likely to miscarry as nonsmokers. Only fourteen percent of the women who miscarried admitted using cocaine, while twenty-nine percent had used cocaine. Cocaine users were one and a half times more likely to miscarry than nonusers.

The good news is millions of people have given up their tobacco habits. Do not wait for a major health crisis such as a heart attack or cancer to inspire you to finally kick the habit. If you are distressed by this addiction, consider it your duty to tell one young person or pregnant woman every day why you wish you had quit at their age. One day, you too will be a successful non-smoker!

> "There is a transcendent power in example.
> We reform others unconsciously, when we walk uprightly."
> —Anne Sophie Swetchine

3 DAY FOOD & ACTIVITY DIARY

	Date:	Date:	Date:
Morning Meal Time:			
Snack			
Noon Meal Time:			
Snack			
Evening Meal Time:			
Snack			
Symptoms (Physical & Emotional)			
Exercise Type & Duration			

Day 10

"We are like tea bags–
we don't know our own strength
until we're in hot water."
—Sister Busche

Green Inside is Clean Inside

When I started my health career in 1974 as a dental hygienist. "Green Inside is Clean Inside" was an excellent slogan I learned from a very health conscious patient. Since then I have discovered a great deal about the life-supporting and healing powers of green foods and chlorophyll.

It is no accident that green plants are vastly abundant on our planet. The chlorophyll in green plants is essential to our health and vitality. It is found in the oceans (algae and seaweeds), in forests, grasslands and agricultural crops.

As plants go through photosynthesis they consume carbon dioxide and produce oxygen, our most important nutrient. Chlorophyll is nearly identical in structure to our body's hemoglobin, which is the compound that carries oxygen through our bloodstream. Where hemoglobin has iron in the center of its molecule, chlorophyll contains magnesium. It is this similar molecular structure that makes chlorophyll an excellent blood cleanser and builder. Chlorophyll is also used by our bodies for wound healing and renewing our blood and tissues. In addition, it has powerful antioxidant and anti-inflammatory properties.

Chlorophyll-rich foods are often deficient in the diets of people who suffer from fatigue. Because green foods are rich in minerals they are usually one of the first things I recommend to build up within individuals who are depleted. The magnesium found in chlorophyll is essential to the production of energy. It activates over three hundred enzymes, including many that are involved in converting carbohydrates, proteins, and fats into ATP, the energy source for every cell in the body. Deficiencies of magnesium can also lead to weakness, depression, irritability, hypoglycemia, sleep disorders, allergies, asthma, constipation, hypertension, fibromyalgia, osteoporosis, migraines, angina and muscle cramps or twitches.

The antioxidant function of plant foods is extremely important in the mitochondria of our cells where we produce energy. The mitochondria provide the energy that drives all of our cellular processes--including nutrient uptake, toxin elimination, and cellular repair. The mitochondria have a DNA that we inherit only from our mothers. This DNA has a different shape (circular) than the twisted, double helical shape of our DNA that determines our genetic features. This shape makes it twenty times more vulnerable to oxidative damage and threatens our ability to produce energy. ***Plant foods are mandatory for protecting our mitochondrial DNA and to preserve energy.***

FOLIC ACID COMES FROM FOLIAGE

Another important reason to consume green foods is the abundance of folic acid, which derives its name from the Latin *folium*, meaning foliage. Folic acid has received a great deal of attention in its role preventing severe birth deformaties such as spina bifida and brain defects. Deficiency of folic acid is also associated with cervical dysplasia, discovered by abnormalities in Pap smear results. It is also a factor in depression, particulaly in the elderly. Folic acid deficiency causes an anemia similar to that of B12, with bigger than normal red blood cells. For this reason, they are often supplemented together.

One of the most significant problems related to folic acid deficiency is with elevated levels of an amino acid, homocysteine, which may lead to coronary artery disease (heart attacks and strokes), cancer and Alzheimer's disease. Since these diseases combined affect the majority of the population, it is evident that we need to eat more green foods.

A great way to improve your energy is to consume daily, foods with high chlorophyll content such as kale, collard greens or dark green salads. Kale is the lovely plant with curly green leaves that is used to decorate salad bars or as plate garnish. Little did you know it was edible! Spinach is also a great source of chlorophyll but frequent consumption needs to be avoided due to its oxalate content which can lead to kidney stones. Unlike spinach, kale and collard greens are usually too dense to eat raw.

Most Americans avoid dark green vegetables because of a slightly bitter flavor yet they are some of the most healing foods available. Unfortunately, the way kale, spinach and collards are often cooked does not enhance their popularity. Most people cook all of the vitality out of these vegetables until they look sloppy, slimy and disgusting. I can remember the childhood trauma of being forced to eat three bites of nasty-tasting spinach as a child at school lunches.

I know this might seem strange but I have coached many patients to eat one of these vegetables at breakfast to give them a roaring start for the day. Every one of my skeptics was amazed at how fast they got their energy back. And because the magnesium in these plants helps improve cellular uptake of glucose by insulin, they can decrease sugar cravings.

When choosing lettuce for salads, always select varieties with the darkest green leaves. The salad greens with a mixture of the different varieties are the best option. Each plant has different phytonutrients that have many healing and antioxidant properties. The mixtures contain some of the more bitter varieties of lettuce that you would not usually eat alone. Skip the "anemic" iceberg lettuce altogether and just focus on leaf lettuces.

Many people who are fatigued tell me they are too tired to cook. Foods that are high in chlorophyll are so simple and fast to prepare that you simply cannot afford to pass them up. These foods are a great place to start and will pay huge dividends in increased energy.

TODAY'S ACTIVITY

ENJOY SOME KALE OR COLLARD GREENS

These are easily found in most grocery stores. They are sold in bunches with about a dozen leaves. Allow one to three leaves per person, depending on size.

1. Wash the leaves thoroughly to remove bugs and dirt.
2. Chop into one inch pieces and boil in salted water for only three to four minutes. The cooking time depends on the time of year. These greens are much more delicate in the spring and require less cooking. In the fall they are much sturdier and may require five minutes of boiling or steaming.
3. Strain and flavor with lemon juice, soy sauce or your favorite salad dressing. In addition to consuming these vegetables alone, they taste great when added to soups and stews.

SUNKEN TREASURES OF CROWN JEWELS

Another class of high-energy green foods is seaweeds or sea vegetables. These foods have been prized since ancient times by people who live along the coasts of Japan, New Zealand, Britain, Ireland and Europe. Because of their rich mineral content, my Macrobiotic mentor, **David Briscoe**, refers to them as the "crown jewels" of the food chain. Most importantly, they are the only decent natural food source of iodine besides shellfish. Iodine deficiency causes low thyroid function, which is a major cause of fatigue. Many varieties are also excellent sources of calcium.

Sea vegetables are very versatile and can be added to soups and salads or cooked with vegetables, beans and grains. They are sold in dehydrated form so a little bit goes a long way. Follow directions on the packages regarding soaking times and preparation. Try to add these to your diet two to three times per week.

Miso soup is an excellent vitality builder that serves as a great way to incorporate sea vegetables. Light or yellow miso is used more for summer soups and the dark barley miso is used in the winter. Dark miso has been aged about eighteen months and has greater health building properties. Use about one half to one teaspoon per cup of liquid and add it just before serving. Do not boil miso. Put a little of the soup broth in a glass measuring cup and mix the miso to soften it. This will allow you to get the clumps out before adding it to the whole pot. Simmer for ten minutes after adding it.

Because sea vegetables often represent new territory for individuals, I have included the following chart to detail by appearance, flavor, and preparation methods, the different varieties of sea vegetables that can be easily incorporated into your diet on a regular basis. For recipes on cooking with sea vegatables, visit David and Cindy Briscoe's web site: **www.macroamerica.com**.

SEA VEGETABLES

- **ARAME** is a delicate and almost sweet sea vegetable that is ideal for beginners. Cook it with carrots and/or onions to enhance its sweetness. It is also good in soups or with tofu. It is rich in calcium and iodine.

- **DULSE** is reddish in color and can be eaten right out of the package. It also is a good match for beginners and children. It has a salty, spicy flavor and works well in salad or stir-fry. It can be fried as an alternative to bacon in a BLT sandwich. Dulse is extremely high in protein, iron, and vitamin B6, and a good source of B12, potassium and fluoride.

- **HIJIKI** is one of the strongest-tasting varieties and not one I would recommend for beginners. It can be sauteed with vegetables or used in soups. It expands up to five times its volume so use it sparingly. Hijiki is an excellent source of calcium and iron.

- **KOMBU** is a wonderful seaweed to boost the flavor of soups, stews, and grains and for tenderizing beans. It is sold in strips that should be washed off and placed into your cooking liquid to soften. Within five minutes, pull it out with tongs, cut it into small pieces and add it back in. If you leave it in its large form it will become very slimy and unappetizing. Kombu is often referred to as "natural MSG" because of its ability to enhance flavors.

- **NORI** is the familiar seaweed you may have seen as the green wrapper around many sushi dishes. It can also be chopped or crumbled to use in soups and salads.

- **WAKAME** is one of my favorite seaweeds. It is most commonly used to make miso soups. It can also be used with vegetables, salads, stir-fry or rice dishes. It is rich in calcium, B vitamins and vitamin C.

GREEN DRINKS

Although I do not believe in coaching people to rely only on health remedies in a bottle, sometimes people will see dramatic progress if they consume one of the "green drink" products available at various health food stores. If you are not yet eating your five servings of vegetables per day it is a good idea to supplement with these. The better ones contain the fat-soluble nutrients, A, E, F, and K, and thus will have a bit of a "gloppy" texture that does not dissolve well in water.

Metagenics has a green phytonutrient product called **Phyto Complete®** that is available in both a powder or tablet form. It contains whole food concentrates of flower pollen extracts, aloe vera, three types of algae, wheat and barley grasses, six different vegetables and the adaptogenic herbs, ginseng, schizandra and astragalus root. It also has tofu powder, rice starch and a variety of other herbs.

In addition, **Metagenics** has a phytonutrient product called **PhytoPhase®** that provides foods and herbs that support healthy liver detoxification, with an emphasis on Phase II enzyme activity discussed in *Day 25--Love Your Liver*. **Dr. Jeffrey Bland** of **The Institute for Functional Medicine**, developed another product supplied by **Metagenics** called **Mitochondrial Resuscitate™**. This formula is designed to provide nutritional support for the proper functioning of the mitochondria for energy production.

Wheat grass juice is another potent revitalizer and detoxifier, and is highly recommended for chronic fatigue. This is available freshly-made at various health food stores and juice bars. If you become a wheat grass enthusiast you can also buy a special device for juicing and easily grow your own plants at home. A small amount goes a very long way. Wheat grass is also available as a powdered "green drink" at health food stores.

Super Blue Green® Algae is a concentrated, wild-crafted food available in powder, capsule or tablet form. This species of algae is known as ***Aphanizomenon flos-aquae***. Unlike **Spirulina** products, which are grown by man, this algae has grown wild for years in a mineral rich lake in Klamath Falls, Oregon. It is harvested every year by the company, **Cell Tech, Inc** (see Resources).

Nutritional values obtained in 1991 indicated that ***Aphanizomenon*** algae had more than twice the content of chlorophyll (300 mg) of **Spirulina** (115mg). I have consumed this product in both the **Omega Sun** and **Alpha Sun** forms since 1995, and credit it for having restored my energy and vitality more than anything else I have used. It is a powerhouse of energy, containing vitamins, minerals and all twenty essential and non-essential amino acids.

Chlorella is another popular algae that has the ability to bind with heavy metals and pesticides and carry them safely out of the body. It also has beneficial effects on the immune system and against carcinogens.

Another important type of algae worth mentioning is ***Dunaliella*** which has more of a reddish brown color. It is the source of beta carotene products and the essential fatty acid DHA, which is often sold in combination with fish oil (EPA/DHA).

HERBAL ENERGY

Products that thrive in the wild have a tremendous healing capacity. This is why there has been such an explosion in the use of wild-crafted herbs and products found growing in the world's rain forests. We cannot afford to destroy the sources of these valuable plants. They are literally God's gift to our health. Their destruction will surely lead to our demise.

Please note: *A popular herb that is on the endangered species list is Golden Seal. It would be prudent to avoid buying products with this ingredient for a few years until it is known to be prolific again.*

A class of plants called adaptogens works on the cellular level to restore energy supplies, increase resistance to disease and infections, boost the immune system and help decrease stress. Studies show that these herbs can heighten energy by increasing oxygen flow to the lungs. The following adaptogens are taken for a month or two with a rest period of a week or more before you resume intake.

HERB	FUNCTION	COMMENTS
American ginseng *(Panax quinquefoliou)*	Increases energy and helps direct internal body fluids to nourish the organs most in need	Cooler and more calming than other ginsengs. Best for people whose body temperatures run hot. Don't use if prone to stomachaches after eating cold foods.
Ashwagandha *(Withania somnifera)*	Aids in restoring muscles, body tissues and bone marrow	Restores adrenal strength. Also used in Indian herbal medicine to improve male libido.
Astragalus *(Astragalus memvranaceus)*	An immune, adrenal and pancreatic tonic	Available as an extract, capsule, tea or in bulk. Avoid if you've had a stroke or have high blood pressure.
Ginger *(Zingiber officinale)*	Anti-inflammatory; eases digestion, improves blood circulation, relieves pain	Best used in winter, since it generates body heat . Can be consumed in everything from soups to stir-fries.
Siberian ginseng *(Eleutherococcus senticosus)*	An immune system stimulant; has a balancing effect on chemicals in the bloodstream, like blood sugar	A powerful adaptogen that helps you cope with stress. Avoid if you have high blood pressure or are taking stimulants. Decreases side effects of chemotherapy.

> **"Common sense is the knack of seeing things as they are, and doing things as they ought to be done."**
> — Josh Billings

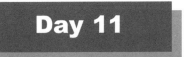

"No pessimist ever discovered the secrets of stars,
or sailed to an uncharted land,
or opened a new heaven to the human spirit."

— Helen Keller

Feeling Pooped?
The answer may be in your colon!

Your intestinal tract plays an important role in your overall health, energy and vitality. A healthy intestinal tract not only allows absorption of nutrients, but also acts as a barrier to keep harmful toxins out of your circulation. It provides the first line of defense as an immune barrier to foreign organisms or toxins that we ingest from our food and water.

Immune function begins with our mouth and tonsils. Next, the extreme acid pH of our stomach acts as a powerful germ killer. It then switches to a strong alkaline pH from our bile and pancreatic enzymes in the small intestine. In addition, we have enormous amounts of approximately four hundred different species of beneficial bacteria throughout our small and large intestines. These bacteria produce compounds that inhibit the growth of various yeast, bacteria and parasites.

Consider the ways we disrupt this environment. An article published in December, 1999 in the **Proceedings of the National Academy of Sciences**, found that our mouths contain nearly five hundred strains of bacteria. Most of them are beneficial germs that digest food and fend off bad germs.

We are indoctrinated into killing bad germs instead of simply supplying good ones to prevent infections. Many people use mouthwash regularly with the expectation that this will kill germs associated with sore throats. However, since this also must kill some of the beneficial bacteria in the mouth, there needs to be a study to discover if this really is a healthy way to decrease the propensity for infections. The recent trend in science is to reconsider our overzealous antibacterial efforts.

Constipation and other colon problems are very common in those whose bacterial flora has been destroyed with frequent or continuous doses of antibiotics. Doctors have incorrectly assumed, for too many years, that your healthy bacterial flora comes back on its own after antibiotic therapy. Even eating yogurt regularly is not enough to regain your flora. Many of the bacteria found in yogurt are not strong enough to persist and implant in your intestines. Taking therapeutic strains of intestinal bacteria, known as probiotics, should be ***obligatory*** during or after every prescription of antibiotics or chemotherapy. Without adequate, healthy bacteria, colon function can either develop constipation or lead to diarrhea, due to bad germs taking over and irritating the lining of the colon. These problems do not always show up immediately. They can take a couple of months to develop.

STOMACH HEALTH

The stomach is one of our most misunderstood organs and is often a target for medications when it is thought to be "misbehaving." Antacids and acid blockers are used extensively in our country without first trying digestive enzymes. Many times enzymes will offer a better solution and prevent the problem from worsening.

Even ulcers have a long history of being incorrectly treated. About ten years ago, **Dr. Barry Marshall** of Australia, discovered a rod-like bacteria when he looked at ulcer tissue under the microscope. He was absolutely certain that most ulcers were caused by this organism, ***Helicobacteria pylori,*** but he was unable to convince his colleagues. Using extreme scientific measures, he inoculated himself with the bacteria, produced the ulcer and then cured himself with the drugs that kill off this germ. In the past ten years, testing for the presence of this germ has become standard procedure for anyone with ulcer symptoms.

Many people, with no obvious ulcers, still suffer from "hyperacidity." This problem often starts with ***inadequate*** hydrochloric acid, which is our primary enzyme for protein digestion. Hydrochloric acid can become low due to aging or a shortage of various nutrients, such as zinc, which is found in a standard multivitamin. When the protein does not digest properly, it literally rots and produces an overabundance of organic acids that are responsible for gastric reflux.

If caught early enough, dietary changes and enzyme supplementation can do wonders for this condition. If you have had this condition for a while and have a significant amount of irritation present, it is not a good idea to start taking hydrochloric acid. This could irritate the condition even further. Ask your doctor or a health food store for a milder plant-based enzyme that works in a low pH range of two to three. You should also take a multivitamin/mineral to encourage your body's own release of hydrochloric acid. Take your enzymes after the meal to allow the release of the body's own enzymes.

COLON FUNCTION

Most people have never discussed their bowel function to any great extent with their doctors. The doctor might ask a question such as, "Any problems with diarrhea or constipation?" If the patient says "No," that is usually the end of the conversation. I often start with questions about a person's frequency and volume of bowel movements. This gives me an idea whether a person's definition of constipation is anything close to mine.

When I explain my definition of normal intestinal function to new patients, I can sense their wide-eyed amazement. Most people assume they have normal function because they have a small amount of daily bowel activity. Later, when their bowel movements are closer to my idea of normal function, they realize proper detoxification and elimination can dramatically improve their fatigue and many other symptoms.

I cannot recall a single patient of mine in eighteen years who has developed colon cancer. There must be something helpful going on with all the vegetables, beneficial bacteria and fiber they have consumed.

In a 1917 *Journal of American Medicine*, **Dr. Kellogg**, of Kellogg's cereal fame, reported that in the treatment of gastrointestinal disease in over forty thousand cases, he had used surgery in only twenty cases. The rest were helped as a result of cleansing the bowels, diet and exercise.

Attention to colon function, and its relation to disease, went "out of vogue" until the 1970's when researchers were studying the Masai tribe in Africa. They found that tribe members who were eating a high fiber, natural diet had an extremely low incidence of appendicitis and all of the typical degenerative diseases common in civilized societies.

When they studied the bowel activity of these people, they found them to have very large diameter stools, much longer in length and more frequent than the typical American or European. This led researchers to start investigating the hazards of a "slow transit time" in bowel function. The longer the waste remains in the colon, the more toxic the bowel environment becomes as well as the greater chance for development of a variety of diseases.

TODAY'S ACTIVITY

HOW IS YOUR INTESTINAL FUNCTION?
Check off the following symptoms that apply to you:

What's normal:

- ❏ Little expansion of belly after meals
- ❏ No abdominal discomfort
- ❏ Bowel movements 2-3 times/day
- ❏ Bowel movements 2-3 feet length/day
- ❏ Diameter of quarter or half dollar
- ❏ Stools sink (unless lots of fiber)
- ❏ Little odor usually
- ❏ Brown color
- ❏ Mild sensation of need to evacuate
- ❏ Short time on the toilet
- ❏ No blood in stools or water
- ❏ No mucus, undigested food

What's abnormal:

- ❏ Bloating, loosening of belt
- ❏ Pain or cramps after eating
- ❏ Constipation/diarrhea
- ❏ Small, hard stools
- ❏ Thin, pencil like stools
- ❏ Stools float (undigested fat)
- ❏ Offensive odor & gas
- ❏ Yellow, gray, green, clay, black
- ❏ Pain, cramping, urgency
- ❏ Reading novels in the bathroom
- ❏ Bloody stools or water
- ❏ Mucus, food, pills visible

If this is an area you need to improve, track your progress on your food and activity diary. At the end of the book you can come back to this chapter and note which "abnormals" are now gone.

PERSONAL STORY

During my childhood, neither of my parents nor our family doctor ever discussed bowel habits. I first discovered the word constipation as a teenager when I was reading a health book looking for causes of my acne. When they listed constipation as one of the causes, I decided to look it up in the dictionary since the word was not familiar to me. Even the dictionary definition was rather vague. I decided to ask my mother. She probably explained that it was when people go longer than a day or so between bowel movements.

Up until that time, I had never noticed how often I had bowel activity, but I knew it was not even close to occurring daily. I decided to pay attention, and lo and behold, I was having bowel movements every seven days! No wonder I had such miserable acne. The plumbing definitely was not eliminating the toxins in the proper route and they were being reabsorbed and excreted through my skin.

We cannot underestimate the value of our intestinal flora. It is said that we literally have more germs in our gut than cells in our entire body. In just **one gram** of stool, scientists have counted 10^{11} bacteria (that's **100 trillion**). Remember that number when you read **Day 13--What's Bugging You?** about some patients I have tested whose stool cultures have *no* beneficial bacteria detected in their stool.

Epidemiological studies indicate a correlation between regular consumption of fermented dairy products and low incidence of colon cancer. Plain yogurt, kefir, cottage cheese and buttermilk are all examples of fermented dairy products that provide beneficial bacteria. However, some dairy companies pasteurize their products after the culturing process is complete, damaging the live bacteria. You can also receive beneficial bacteria by consuming tempeh (fermented soy) or sauerkraut. The following chart lists the many important benefits of our bacterial flora.

FUNCTIONS OF BENEFICIAL BACTERIA FLORA

- Synthesize vitamins (B2, B5, B6, B12, biotin, K)
- Aid digestion
- Sweeten breath
- Improve bowel regularity
- Enhance natural immunity (sixty percent of immune function happens in the gut because that is where we interface with the outside world)
- Inhibit the growth of unfriendly bacteria and yeast
- Help metabolize cholesterol and reproductive hormones
- Control the pH of the colon
- Short chain fatty acid (SCFA) production
    --Produced by bacterial fermentation of water soluble fiber
    --Preferred fuel of colon lining cells = growth factor for a healthy colon
    --Controls fluid balance in colon (fermentation of fiber releases water)

Therapeutic grade bacterial products sold to restore natural flora are known as probiotics, which literally means, "promotes life." It is the opposite of the word antibiotic, meaning "against life." The two most prolific beneficial bacteria in our gut are **Lactobacillus acidophilus** and **Bifidobacterium**. The species, **Bifidobacterium infantis**, is the first flora to colonize the intestines of newborns. With that in mind, if an infant is given antibiotics, this is the only species that should be given to restore flora until the child is eighteen months of age. This will prevent diaper rash and the mouth yeast infection known as "Thrush."

The kind of acidophilus I use in my practice is called **NCFM™**, which is a human strain developed by the **North Carolina Food & Microbiology Group**. It is supplied by **Metagenics** in a product called **Ultra Dophilus®** and in combination with Bifidus bacteria in a product called **Ultra Flora Plus®.** The **NCFM™** species is proven to survive stomach acid and bile and adhere to the intestinal tract.

Another benefit of **Metagenics** brand acidophilus and bifidus products is the ability to buy them in a powder form rather than capsules. It is not only less expensive that way, but drinking it down with water allows you to inoculate healthy bacteria throughout your mouth, tonsils and throat. This may be an important preventive factor in gingivitis, mouth ulcers, sore throats, sinusitis and ear infections.

PROPERTIES OF THE NCFM™ STRAIN OF LACTOBACILLUS ACIDOPHILUS

- Human strain developed by the North Carolina Food & Microbiology Group
- Survives in the human digestive tract
- Adheres to human intestinal cells
- Produces natural antimicrobial (germ killing) substances such as lactic acid, hydrogen peroxide, and possibly acetic and benzoic acids
- Stimulates immunity
- Prevents/improves infectious diarrhea
- Improves small bowel bacterial overgrowth
- Improves lactose digestion in humans
- Detoxifies the bowel
- Assimilates cholesterol and decreases serum cholesterol
- Improves neurological symptoms in kidney dialysis patients
- Inhibits enzymes such as beta-glucuronidase and nitroreductase that induce colon cancer
- Suitable as a probiotic for the urogenital (urinary/vaginal) tract

---

Unfortunately, many lactating women do not produce **Bifidus** bacteria in their milk, leaving the child more vulnerable to infection. Both **acidophilus** and **bifidus** bacteria should be supplemented in pregnant women to ensure establishment of normal flora in the child. This is especially important since yeast overgrowth in the vagina is very common during pregnancy, and the baby will be exposed to that yeast during the birthing process.

Supplementation of **Bifidus infantis** can be accomplished by adding about one eighth teaspoon or less of the powder to bottles of breast milk or formula. Or, a mother can just put a clean, wet finger in the bottle of **Bifidus** powder and let the baby lick it off her finger. I trust **Metagenics** brand of **Bifidus infantis** for infants because I know they are very diligent about ensuring that their products are free of contaminants. A 1990 study of eleven brands of bacteria products in the **Journal of Obstetrics and Gynecology** found **ten** of the eleven brands tested contained a contaminant.

Purity of probiotics is also important when inserting them rectally or vaginally in enemas or douches. Many of my patients have used these techniques to provide faster relief from itching.

PROPERTIES OF *BIFIDOBACTERIA*

- Lowers blood cholesterol levels
- Reduces blood ammonia levels which detoxifies the bowel and reduces toxic burden to the liver
- Inhibits the growth of potential pathogens (disease-causing germs) by producing short-chain fatty acids (SCFA's) such as acetate, lactate, propionate, butyrate and formate. The most plentiful SCFA acetate inhibits yeasts, molds and bacteria.
- Restores the normal intestinal flora during antibiotic therapy - creates the proper environment for all bacteria to reappear
- Produces vitamins
- Acts as immunomodulators (e.g. promotes attack against malignant cells and unfriendly microorganisms)
- A breast-fed infant has approximately ninety-nine percent *Bifidus infantis* species. This is the only bacteria species that should be supplemented for infants until age eighteen months.
- *Bifidus* remains the predominant beneficial bacteria throughout life.
- Decreased *Bifidus* in the stool is a sign of aging and ill health.

WHAT DO ABNORMAL INTESTINAL SYMPTOMS MEAN?

The reason your abdomen bloats after eating is usually one of three things. If you are not producing enough stomach acid, your belly will often bloat immediately after eating. If it occurs one to two hours later it can relate to inadequate bile salts or pancreatic enzymes. It can also be caused by eating an abundance of sugar, alcohol, or flour products which are feeding excessive yeast. The yeast ferments the simple carbohydrates and gives off carbon dioxide and other gases. If you have ever baked bread, recall how you give sugar to yeast and then the yeast produces gas that allows the dough to rise.

Pain and cramping symptoms can be due to lactose intolerance, gluten intolerance or other food allergies. It can also be due to harmful germs in your gut interacting with the foods or inflaming your intestines. **Day 13-- What's Bugging You?** will cover some of the different germs found in stool cultures.

Constipation can occur even if a person is having a daily bowel movement. When a person is having good bowel activity they are expelling two to three feet of bowel movement per day. Two to six-inch bowel movements are not adequate. You will see a major improvement in your energy when your bowels are eliminating properly.

A combination of **both** fiber and bacterial probiotics are necessary to get the bowel working more efficiently. Either one alone will not do the trick. Those who are not getting enough fiber in their diets should supplement it, because sluggish bowel transit time is a major risk factor for colon cancer and other degenerative diseases.

Most people are familiar with psyllium-based fiber products, but usually that is not my first choice for someone with constipation. Many people with constipation feel worse after taking psyllium, either due to an allergy, or because it sometimes dries out their bowel further and feels like concrete.

Metagenics has a hypoallergenic fiber product called **UltraFiber™**, which I have found to be effective and well tolerated for constipation problems involving small, hard stools. This fiber gets fermented by our healthy intestinal bacteria to produce a short chain fatty acid (SCFA) called n-butyrate. This SCFA nourishes our bowel and adds valuable water. This is the primary means to get moisture back in the bowel. I have had numerous patients become terribly frustrated because their attempts at drinking lots of water did nothing for their colon dryness.

After a patient gets the moisture back, I might add a psyllium fiber if they are still troubled by thin, pencil-like stools. I usually recommend they take one type of fiber in the morning and the other type at bedtime. Thin stools are an important symptom to correct. If they persist you should have a colonoscopy to rule out a tumor occupying space in the colon.

Both types of fiber should be added slowly, such as a half scoop per day to start. They can be mixed with water or other beverages, and should be taken at the same time as bacteria products. Neither of **Metagenics'** fiber products contains sugar or artificial sweeteners. Their psyllium product is called **UltraBalance Herbulk®**.

Floating stools can occur if you are taking a lot of fiber. Another common reason for floating stools is the inability to digest fat properly. The fat passes into your stool and floats just like a bar of soap. One of the first phases of fat digestion is the release of bile salts. These are produced by the liver and stored in the gall bladder. I call bile salts the "liquid dishwashing soap of our intestinal tract." They emulsify our fats so they can be properly absorbed.

Sometimes people do not produce adequate bile, or they have difficulties after their gall bladder is removed and need supplementation. I frequently recommend **Cholocol®** bile salts from **Standard Process Labs** (see Resources) or their other product, **A-F Betafood®**, which thins out the bile and allows it to flow better. **Lipo-Gen™** by **Metagenics** will also help with bile function.

Another reason for poor fat digestion occurs when you drink ice cold beverages with meals. Cold interferes with the release of digestive enzymes and the ability of fats to properly dissolve. I explain it to my patients this way:

"Imagine trying to wash greasy dishes in cold dishwater." This is why you must use only room temperature or hot beverages when drinking with a meal.

For most Asians, meals start with hot soup to set the proper environment for digestion. Hot tea is also served with or after meals. Have you ever noticed how common it is to feel bloated after eating Mexican food? It is not that Mexican food is any harder to digest. The bloating is usually caused when digestion is hindered by washing down chips and salsa with ample quantities of cold beverages prior to the main meal.

It is possible to decrease the offensive odor from stools or gas by figuring out the source. It can be produced when you have inadequate digestive enzymes, poor bile production, or from gases produced by various germs in your intestines. ***Day 13--What's Bugging You?*** will discuss how to identify and treat organisms that produce offensive gas.

Yellow, gray, green or clay colored stools can be a sign of liver or gall bladder dysfunction. Black stools are a sign of bleeding high in the digestive tract such as the stomach, duodenum or esophagus. The blood turns black from the action of digestive enzymes on the blood. Blood in stools or dripping into the toilet relates to bleeding either in the colon or from hemmorrhoids. Blood can also come from extreme inflammation of the colon, such as with ulcerative colitis. Colon cancer lesions often discharge only a small amount of blood that is too minute to be seen with the naked eye. This blood is detected by the Hemoccult tests given by doctors to perform at home.

Pain, cramping or urgency related to evacuation indicates that some irritant is triggering a hyper-response to peristalsis. I have seen this associated with sensitivity to foods or from an overabundance of harmful germs or yeasts.

Mucus in the stools can be a sign of intestinal inflammation. It can also come about from the action of fiber or bentonite products adsorbing excessive mucus in the intestinal tract. An overabundance of mucus-causing foods, such as dairy and flour products, contribute to this problem. Food and pills visible in the stool relate to inadequate digestive enzyme activity or from the pill having an indigestible, hard coating. Some vitamins use a coating made from the shells of insects.

Hopefully, this information will give you a greater awareness of how to achieve more normal bowel function and encourage you to seek the advice of a doctor when abnormal signs persist. Intestinal problems are much easier to treat when they are detected early. **Katie Couric** of the ***Today Show*** cautions those who might put off going to the doctor with colon problems, "Don't die of embarrassment!"

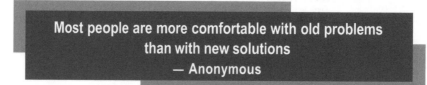

Most people are more comfortable with old problems
than with new solutions
— Anonymous

Day 12

"Energy is the power that drives every human being. It is not lost by exertion but maintained by it."

— Germaine Green

Take a Walk, Skip, or a Jump!

Exercise is absolutely essential to your health. It is a great way to build oxygen, assist with detoxification and reduce stress. **Dr. C. Norman Shealy**, author of ***90 Days to Self-Health***, once made the statement, "Inactivity is one of the most harmful forms of stress." In order to build your energy and vitality, you must engage in a variety of activities that you will enjoy doing regularly.

If you are presently inactive, now is the time to get started on some sort of daily exercise or recreation. Even if you are chronically ill, you can find some easy forms of movement that will not exhaust you. It is best to first discuss with your doctor the activities that are best suited for your present state of health.

Be realistic about choosing a time of day when you will be most successful at consistently exercising. Do not plan to do your exercise at the end of the day if you are typically too exhausted at that time. Nine times out of ten you will talk yourself out of it.

If you have started and stopped exercise programs several times before, begin with a small time commitment, such as ten or fifteen minutes. Avoid rationalizing that you are depriving yourself of fifteen minutes of productivity in your workday. Those fifteen minutes will translate into at least an extra hour or more of productivity that you presently spend in the "Twilight Zone."

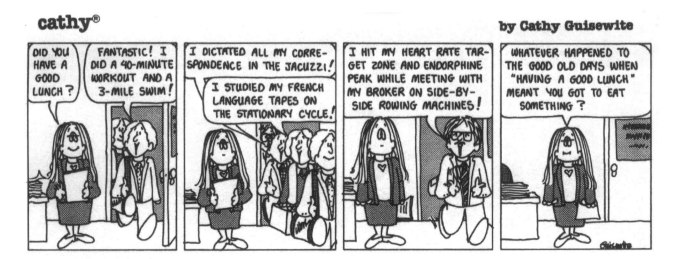

TYPES OF EXERCISE

Short walks, simple yoga stretches and Tai Chi exercises are usually well-tolerated and good energy-builders. Be sure to call the class instructor to find out the pace of the class to determine if it is compatible with your tolerance for exercise.

Although it may seem too difficult for an inactive person, a mountain bike is a wonderful exercise device for beginners. It is very simple to shift gears and can easily be ridden by anyone on flat terrain. If you have weak legs you can downshift to make pedalling effortless to pedal. A mountain bike does not have the balance difficulties of a low handlebar, touring bike and therefore can be used by all ages. For those recovering from chronic illness, it is nice to be able to mix up pedaling and coasting so you only have to do short bursts of activity. Most bikes now have twenty-one gears, allowing you to easily change your pace as you get stronger.

The most valuable benefit of a mountain bike is the psychological boost that comes from becoming more mobile and covering more territory. Walking over a small area can become very boring and discouraging. It is also wonderful to feel the cool breeze a bike offers to prevent becoming overheated. If you are apprehensive about whether you will feel comfortable on a bike, many bike shops will allow you to take one for a "test drive" before buying.

The improvement of fatigue, insomnia and depression from exercise is almost immediate. Walking outdoors has the added benefit of improving seasonal affective disorder (SAD) caused by the light deprivation of the winter months. To receive the greatest benefit for SAD, you must walk in the early morning without glasses or contacts to nourish the pineal gland and activate melatonin. If it is impossible for you to walk without corrective lenses, spend an extra ten minutes sitting outside doing breathing exercises with your lenses off, eyes open and no sunglasses.

Resist the temptation to clutter your mind with tapes or music while you walk. The action of our gait during walking is very balancing to the nervous system. Avoid overloading your senses with extra stimuli. Some of your best ideas and problem solving abilities will come during walks.

Many towns have swimming pool classes for people with a variety of conditions such as arthritis or multiple sclerosis. Water provides wonderful buoyancy and avoids overheating of painful joints.

If you prefer to exercise at home you can obtain one of the popular mini-trampolines that are about four feet in diameter. These are very inexpensive, light-weight and easy to roll into a corner after use. If you have a low tolerance for exercise, just slightly lift your heels to get a gentle bouncing action. This particular exercise device is one of the best for moving stagnant lymph fluid through our bodies.

When you are just getting started with an exercise program, resist becoming frustrated if you can only tolerate three to five minutes of activity. We all have to start with our own capabilities. Pay attention to how your body feels to prevent exhaustion or strain. Remember, most marathon runners probably started their first running program with just one mile. Most of them could not even run 10 miles for quite awhile. Sign up for some 5K runs that encourage walkers. It will be inspiring to discover how many people are struggling to go the distance.

Consider ways to increase activity in your daily life. Use stairs instead of elevators. Park farther away from the door and walk. Bike when going for lunch or on errands. Teach your children that bicycles are a valuable form of transportation. Encourage your town or state to pave an extra few feet for bike paths along the road.

PERSONAL STORY

The frustration and hassles of using busy streets for biking caused me to make bike paths a high priority when choosing a town for our recent relocation to Colorado. Our city recognizes the importance of the bicycle as a means of transportation because of the large number of college students and school-age children who bike to school. It certainly saves on bus expenses. My son's high school requires every teen within two miles to bike or walk to school. This is a great daily exercise that helps fill in the gaps for cutbacks in physical education classes in our schools. Obesity in children is becoming rampant and they could benefit from more opportunities to walk or bike.

MORE VIGOROUS ACTIVITY

Dancing is another wonderful activity that has been enjoyed in nearly every country since ancient times. Have you ever seen a dancer who was not smiling? Many towns offer classes on country, folk, and ethnic dances that require no partners.

Jumping rope is a good exercise for those winter indoor days. This exercise is only for someone who is in good shape and already capable of running at least one mile. It should be avoided if you have problems with your knees and feet or suffer from spinal or hip pains. Start out with short one minute sessions and increase your time slowly.

It is best to only jump rope for three minutes at a time, with a one-minute rest period between intervals. To avoid injuries, do not exceed a maximum of nine minutes total to avoid injuries. Many athletes only skip rope for about six weeks and then refrain for a period of one month. When you choose to resume this activity, return to the one-minute level and work back up again.

Many athletic trainers recommend changing your workout every four to six weeks. This will prevent plateaus and boredom. Write the activities in your diet and activity journal to monitor your progress. You may also want to take before-and-after measurements of your chest, waist, hips, and thighs to more accurately observe changes.

PULSE RATE

Monitoring your pulse rate while exercising is very important to prevent over-training. Exercising at a level over your maximum pulse rate is not only dangerous to your heart but can also exhaust your adrenal glands, weaken your immune system and make you more prone to injury. Aerobic activity ideally burns fat for energy. Running too fast for long periods of time puts your body into anaerobic metabolism. Instead of burning fat, this causes your body to burn glucose (which is in very short supply) and can lead to a variety of health problems.

TODAY'S ACTIVITY

TESTING YOUR PULSE

Test your pulse upon awakening or after you have been resting in a chair for at least ten minutes. Take three fingers (with the index being #1) and place them either on the front side of your neck or on the inside of the wrist on the same side as your thumb. Soon you will start to detect your pulse under your fingertips. Take your pulse for fifteen seconds and multiply that number by four to get your rate for one minute.

For example, 20 beats x 4 = 80 beats/minute.

Your pulse: _____ beats/minute.

This is your resting pulse rate or heart rate. Average values for adults are 60 – 80 beats per minute (bpm). Well-trained athletes can have pulse rates around 50 bpm. Newborns can have a pulse rate of 70 – 170 bpm. By age four the average heart rate is 70 – 115 bpm.

The **American Heart Association** considers a normal resting pulse rate for adult men and women to be anywhere from 50 to 100 bpm. New evidence suggests that elevations of pulse rate within this normal range strongly predict an increased risk of dying, rather than recovering, from a heart attack.

PULSE RATE AS A PREDICTOR OF CARDIOVASCULAR DEATHS

The following information was taken from the May, 1999 issue of ***Alternatives™ For The Health Conscious Individual***, by **Dr. David Williams**. Reprinted by permission. For more information on Dr. David Williams' monthly newsletter, please call (800) 527-3044.

Doctors at the Italian **University of Padova** released a study in 1999, which tracked 763 men and 1,175 women, aged sixty-five and older for a period of twelve years. They found an elevated resting heart rate appeared to be a strong predictor of cardiovascular-related deaths in men. This included deaths from heart attack, stroke, congestive heart failure, and kidney failure. The research did not show as strong a correlation with women.

The research subjects were divided into five different groups based on their resting heart rates. Among the men, those in the highest fifth (over eighty heartbeats per minute) had almost three times the risk of cardiovascular-related death compared to those in the group with the lowest heart rates.

Even after the researchers made adjustments for known cardiovascular disease risk factors, those in the top fifth of the group still had almost double the risk of dying compared to the bottom fifth of the group. (***Archives of Internal Medicine*** 99;159 (6):585-92)

This study confirms heart rate research conducted in England, Germany, and the United States. Compare your resting pulse rate to the chart below to see how you compare to this recent research. Although this research has been most applicable to men, further studies with larger groups may suggest that women would also benefit from these guidelines.

CARDIVASCULAR RISK LEVELS FOR MEN BASED ON RESTING HEART RATE

Below 64 Beats per minute = in the healthy range

64 to 69 beats per minute = Mild risk

70 to 75 beats per minute = Moderate risk

Over 76 beats per minute = high risk

If you are at moderate to high risk, consider this a valuable early warning tool to inform you whether you are putting enough emphasis on decreasing your cardiac risk factors. Consider those things you can control today, such as eliminating caffeine (stimulants), eating more vegetables, less junk foods, leaner and smaller quantities of meats, exercising more, and employing stress reduction habits such as breathing exercises, biofeedback, anger management, and stretching exercises.

Start working to eliminate the obvious cardiac risk factors such as obesity, smoking, excessive alcohol intake, high blood pressure and abnormal cholesterol levels. Heart attacks may be the leading cause of death but they are also the most preventable major health problem.

Be sure you protect your heart with the "Big 3" nutritional categories: multivitamin/minerals, antioxidants, and omega-3 fats. In addition, you might consider discussing with a holistic physician whether you need to add magnesium, taurine, garlic, coenzyme Q-10, hawthorn berry or l-carnitine to your nutrient regime.

EXERCISE PULSE RATES

There have been numerous formulas for determining maximum exercise heart rate. An easy method is to subtract your age from 180. Therefore, a forty-year-old person has a maximum rate of 140. If a person has chronic diseases such as asthma or heart disease they should decrease the rate by another five or ten points for *each* condition, based on severity.

When taking your pulse while exercising, take it for only *six* seconds and multiply it by ten. Therefore, a person trying to not go over 140 bpm should have a maximum six second pulse rate of fourteen. Another way to tell if you are exercising too strenuously is if it is difficult to talk during your activity. You should not experience difficulty breathing during exercise. If lowering the intensity does not alleviate breathing difficulties, contact your doctor.

PULSE RECOVERY AFTER EXERCISE

Another important discovery about pulse rates was reported by researchers at the **Cleveland Clinic**, in the October 28, 1999 issue of the ***New England Journal of Medicine***. The discovery occured while doing routine treadmill tests. They found that the rate at which the heartbeat slows, after someone exercises to exhaustion and stops, can help doctors spot those patients needing aggressive treatment to prevent heart attacks.

Normally, when someone exercises to exhaustion and then stops, the heart rate drops fifteen to twenty-five bpm within one minute. **Dr. Michael Lauer** and his colleagues found that for patients whose heart rate fell less than twelve beats one minute after exercising, the risk of dying within six years was ***four times greater*** than for those with a healthy heart.

If you are presently using a treadmill or doing any other form of strenuous exercise you can try this test yourself. If you are going to your doctor for a stress test, be sure to ask them to include this extra pulse measurement one minute after the conclusion of the test.

Keeping your exercise heart rate under the proper level and discovering how well your heart recovers after exercise may prevent tragic heart attacks after exercising. A famous example of this was **James Fixx**, a well-known writer on the benefits of running, who died while running in 1984.

Becoming aware of your pulse rate is just as important as knowing your blood pressure is within normal limits. Keep track of a few readings. Test it under various circumstances such as after a cup of coffee or soda, after driving home in busy traffic, or after an emotional stress. If you suffer from allergies or asthma, you may also want to test your pulse before and after meals. Some doctors believe a large increase in the pulse after eating could indicate an allergy to some of the foods.

TODAY'S ACTIVITY

Take some opportunities today to check your pulse rate under various conditions:

Pulse: Circumstances:

_____

_____

   Remember to keep track of your daily exercise on your Food and Activity Diaries. You may also want to include your pulse rates on the charts at various times. If your pulse rate consistently runs over ninety be sure to track down the cause. Eliminate caffeine or stimulatory herbs such as Ma huang, and illegal drugs such as cocaine and methamphetamines.

   Do not stop any prescription drugs without consulting your doctor. If you are taking asthma drugs, Ritalin or other stimulatory medications, you may want to keep track of your pulse rate and discuss it with your doctor. If you cannot find the source of your high pulse rate, or if your pulse rate fails to fall twelve beats within one minute after exercising, contact your doctor.

"Power is the faculty or capacity to act, the strength and potency to accomplish something. It is the vital energy to make choices and decisions. It also includes the capacity to overcome deeply embedded habits and to cultivate higher, more effective ones."
— Stephen R. Covey

3 DAY FOOD & ACTIVITY DIARY

	Date:	Date:	Date:
Morning Meal Time:			
Snack			
Noon Meal Time:			
Snack			
Evening Meal Time:			
Snack			
Symptoms (Physical & Emotional)			
Exercise Type & Duration			

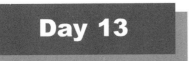

"The only way to be who you want to be
is by being what you haven't been."

—Sally Edwards

What's Bugging You?

In the mid-1980's, doctors **William Crook**, **Orian Truss** and **John Trowbridge** published extremely popular books about how our health can become severely impacted by excessive intestinal overgrowth of a yeast normally found in our gut called ***Candida albicans.*** This yeast imbalance creates an entire constellation of symptoms that can affect our intestines, energy, brain function, emotions, sinuses, lungs, vaginal area, urinary tract, etc.

Since that time we have learned that many other organisms, besides yeast, can colonize the gastrointestinal tract and create dysfunction there and throughout the body. Instead of calling everything of this nature a "candida problem," we now refer to this as dysbiosis, which essentially means "bad way of life." You can also think of it more easily as "bad germs." **Leo Galland, M.D**., coined this term and has written several books and papers on the subject.

Dysbiosis refers to the condition where a bad diet, various drugs and lifestyle imbalances have disrupted the normal and healthy population of beneficial bacteria in the intestines. This leaves it open to the overgrowth of yeast, fungi, parasites and potentially harmful strains of bacteria. This intestinal imbalance, in turn, adversely affects other important organ systems via toxic stress and by interfering with nutrient absorption and utilization.

According to a recent survey of more than 2,500 households, digestive problems such as bloating, abdominal pain, and diarrhea are much more common than previously thought. Researchers from the **University of North Carolina** and **John Hopkins University** found that more than forty percent of American adults reported suffering at least one of these symptoms in the past month.

About three-fourths of the respondents who reported bloating or distension, rated their symptoms as moderate or severe. The need to reduce their normal activities by at least one-half due to their digestive complaints was reported by ten percent. Nearly twice as many women than men reported diarrhea and bloating on more than eleven days in the past month. From forty to sixty percent of the respondents took medication for their gastrointestinal symptoms.

Each year, colorectal cancer claims over fifty thousand lives in the U.S. alone. It is now the second most common cause of cancer-related deaths worldwide. Improving the screening process is critical for making inroads against this disease, which some researchers are now calling the "major preventable healthcare problem in the U.S."

Identifying and treating the reasons for colon dysfunction and dysbiosis are the major ways to prevent a sick colon from turning into a deadly colon. This chapter will explore a vastly underutilized method of colon diagnosis that is an excellent tool for helping the physician restore health and vitality to prevent or reverse disease.

The following dysbiosis questionnaire should help you and your physician evaluate the possible role of dysbiosis in contributing to your health problems. However, it will not provide an automatic "Yes" or "No" answer. The questionnaire is designed for adults, so the scoring system will not be as applicable for children. Scores for women will run higher because more items in this quiz apply exclusively to women.

In my practice, I have seen several people with scores over four hundred because they are so ill and toxic they have nearly every symptom on the list. These people are severely fatigued and have a very low quality of life. It is extremely gratifying when the majority of those symptoms abate after their dysbiosis is brought under control.

Case Study

"Susan" was a patient suffering from severe constipation, fatigue, headaches, backaches and irritability. Her initial Dysbiosis score was 405 and her Toxicity Quiz score was 110. She had a stool culture test that showed two harmful germs: a 2+ score on **Candida albicans** and a 1+ on a bacteria called **Citrobacter freundii**. Even though 4+ is considered the worst-case scenario, her health was still being significantly impacted by these organisms. The inability to discharge them and other toxins through normal bowel activity was causing many severe symptoms.

Six weeks later, after taking the necessary drugs and nutrients and reestablishing normal bowel function, "Susan's" scores improved dramatically. Her Dysbiosis score decreased to 141 and her Toxicity score was thirty-nine.

	Before	After
Dysbiosis Score	405	141
Toxicity Score	110	39

The following questionnaire was adapted from **Dr. William G. Crook's** book, *Tired-So Tired and the "Yeast Connection."* He has several books available on his website, **www.candida-yeast.com** or by calling (800) 227-2627.

TODAY'S ACTIVITY

DYSBIOSIS QUESTIONNAIRE & SCORE SHEET

For each question you answer "Yes," circle the Point Score. Total your score and record it in the box at the end of the section. Then move on to Sections B and C and score as directed.

Section A: History   ***Point Score***

1. Have you taken antibiotics for skin, acne or anything else, for one month (or longer)? _ _ _ _ _ _ 25
2. Have you, ***at any time in your life,*** taken other "broad spectrum" antibiotics for respiratory, urinary or other infections for two months or longer, or in short courses four or more times in a 1 year period? _ 20
3. Have you taken a broad spectrum antibiotic drug – even a single course? _ _ _ _ _ _ _ _ _ _ 6
4. Have you, at any time in your life, been bothered by recurrent or persistent prostatitis, vaginitis or other problems affecting your reproductive organs? _ _ _ _ _ _ _ _ _ _ _ _ _ _ _ 25
5. Have you taken birth control pills or shots (DepoProvera)
   For more than 5 years? _ 25
   For more than 2 years? _ 15
   For 6 months to 2 years? _ 8
6. Have you been pregnant
   1 time? _ 3
   2 or more times? _ 5
7. Have you taken prednisone, Decadron or other cortisone-type drug:
   For more than 6 months? _ 25
   For more than 2 weeks? _ 15
   For 2 weeks or less? _ 6
8. Does exposure to perfumes, insecticides, fabric shop odors and other chemicals provoke:
   Moderate to severe symptoms? _ 20
   Mild symptoms? _ 5
9. Are your symptoms worse on damp, muggy days or in moldy places? _ _ _ _ _ _ _ _ _ _ _ _ 20
10. Have you had athlete's foot, ring worm, "jock itch" or other chronic fungus infections of the skin or nails?
    Mild to moderate? _ 10
    Severe or persistant? _ 20
11. Do you crave sugar? _ 10
12. Do you crave breads? _ 10
13. Do you crave alcoholic beverages? _ 10
14. Does tobacco smoke ***really*** bother you? _ 10
15. Have you ever had parasitic infection, dysentery or unexplained episode of prolonged diarrhea and/or intestinal distress? _ 15
16. Have you ever consumed chlorinated (or chemically treated) drinking water for 3 or more months? _ 15
17. Do you consume commercially raised meat or poultry (antibiotic fed) on a regular basis? _ _ _ _ 15
18. Do you eat processed foods regularly? _ 20
19. Do you drink alcohol or consume coffee daily? _ _ _ _ _ _ _ _ _ _ _ _ _ _ _ _ _ 20
20. Have you ever had an ulcer, colitis, Crohn's disease or diverticulitis? _ _ _ _ _ _ _ _ _ _ _ 35
21. Were you breast fed?
    If yes, but for less than 3 months _ 20
    If no _ 35

Total Score, Section A _____

TODAY'S ACTIVITY CONTINUED

For the next 2 sections, enter the appropriate figure in the Point Score column:

Occasional or mild symptoms 3
Frequent &/or moderately severe ... 6
Severe or disabling symptoms 9

Add the total score and record it in the box at the end of this section.

Section B: Major Symptoms

Point Score

1. Fatigue or lethargy ____
2. Feeling of being "drained" ____
3. Poor memory ____
4. Feeling "spacey" or "unreal" ____
5. Depression ____
6. Numbness, burning or tingling ____
7. Muscle aches ____
8. Muscle weakness or paralysis ____
9. Pain and/or swelling in joints ____
10. Abdominal pain ____
11. Constipation ____
12. Diarrhea ____
13. Bloating ____
14. Troublesome vaginal discharge ____
15. Persistent vaginal burning ____

16. Persistent vaginal itch ____
17. Prostatitis ____
18. Impotence ____
19. Loss of sexual desire ____
20. Endometriosis ____
21. Cramps and/or other menstrual irregularities ____
22. Premenstrual tension ____
23. Spots in front of eyes ____
24. Erratic vision ____
25. Eczema, dermatitis, psoriasis ____

Total Score, Section B _____

Section C: Other Symptoms *Point Score*

1. Drowsiness ____
2. Irritability or jitteriness ____
3. Incoordination ____
4. Inability to concentrate ____
5. Frequent mood swings ____
6. Headaches ____
7. Dizziness/loss of balance ____
8. Pressure above ears, feeling of head swelling & tingling ____
9. Itching ____
10. Other rashes ____
11. Heartburn ____
12. Indigestion ____
13. Belching and intestinal gas ____
14. Mucus in stools ____
15. Hemorrhoids ____
16. Dry mouth ____
17. Rash or blisters in mouth ____
18. Bad breath ____

19. Nasal congestion or discharge ____
20. Joint swelling or arthritis ____
21. Postnasal drip ____
22. Nasal itching ____
23. Sore or dry throat ____
24. Cough ____
25. Pain or tightness in chest ____
26. Wheezing/shortness of breath ____
27. Urinary urgency or frequency ____
28. Burning on urination ____
29. Failing vision ____
30. Burning or tearing of eyes ____
31. Recurrent infection/fluid in ears ____
32. Ear pain or hearing loss ____

Total Score, Section C _____
Total Score, Section A _____
Total Score, Section B _____

GRAND TOTAL SCORE [ ]

Adapted from **W.G. Crook**, *Tired-So Tired!* and *The Yeast Connection*, Professional Books, 2001.
Used with permission.

Interpretation	Women	Men
• Dysbiosis related health problems are *almost certainly* present	>180	>140
• Dysbiosis related health problems are *probably* present	120-180	80-140
• Dysbiosis related health problems are *possibly* present	60-119	40-89
• Dysbiosis related health problems are *less likely* present	<60	<40

STOOL CULTURE TESTS

In the 1980's, two naturapathic doctors in North Carolina decided to start experimenting with laboratory analysis of the stool to determine what was normal function and what was present in people with various health problems. This experimentation evolved into a test called the **Comprehensive Digestive Stool Analysis**. It measures various parameters of intestinal function including a culture of bacteria and yeast present. It can also be expanded to include a parasitology test.

This one test evolved into an entire laboratory that now employs more than 250 people and serves over ten thousand doctors in twenty-seven countries. Their name is **Great Smokies Diagnostic Laboratory** and they now do 125 different lab tests on blood, urine, stools, saliva and hair.

The **Comprehensive Digestive Stool Analysis (CDSA)** is a very simple test of a single stool sample. It is collected at home, with no preparation necessary except for the prior avoidance of certain drugs or nutritional products such as enzymes and vitamin C for about three days prior to the test. I also recommend my clients stop taking bacteria supplements and fiber products for the same length of time.

The **CDSA** measures thirteen different parameters of digestive function, including digestion, absorption, metabolic markers for colon regeneration and detoxification abnormalities, beneficial bacteria, additional bacteria which may cause disease, yeast and pH (acid or alkaline balance).

We now know the various symptoms originally attributed to yeast imbalances can actually be caused by a variety of bacteria, parasites and often a much broader selection of yeast than just the ***Candida albicans*** species. The information gathered from the stool analysis allows a doctor to select a treatment that accurately targets the specific offending germs and other present abnormalities.

To determine the most effective treatment for harmful germs or excessive yeasts, **Great Smokies** does a ***culture and sensitivity test*** on the patient's own germ. This identifies which drugs or natural products are most inhibitory to the organism. This puts an end to the "try this, try that" parade of drugs and other nutritional remedies patients and their doctors often experiment with to try to alleviate their symptoms.

In many cases, the overgrowth of germs in the intestines is the source for recurrent infections in the vagina, urinary tract, sinuses, etc. This test is an extremely valuable way to more permanently get the offending organism under control. The colon is a six foot long tube with a great environment for bad germs to flourish.

Think of the colon as a gigantic dormitory with the vagina, bladder or sinuses being just one room of the dorm. This is why doctors treat vaginitis, cystitis and sinusitis until they are blue in the face and these problems just keep returning. However, when you improve the health of the colon these smaller areas become healthier as well.

When a **CDSA** indicates a drug therapy is the most effective treatment, I send the patient to medical doctors who are familiar with this test. They often treat them for longer than a week to ensure sufficient decrease or eradication of the germ. The typical course of treatment with many drugs can last two to four weeks.

Since drugs can be both expensive and toxic to the liver, you need to be sure you are using the correct one. **Great Smokies'** *culture and sensitivity tests* help identify the right therapy for the germ. These tests also give you the option of knowing whether a less toxic natural product will do the job.

The following are some interesting cases that show you the value of this test with a variety of health problems, all involving fatigue.

CASE 1

This case taught me many types of yeast are often too tenacious to kill off with natural remedies. This was a fifty-nine-year-old woman who suffered from severe diarrhea, with eight to ten watery bowel movements per day, for over a year. She had been to a family doctor, GI specialist, Chinese herbalist, and tried every remedy I knew.

She first declined to have this test done because she did not want to spend the money. I finally convinced her that she had spent well over the cost of the test on the various drugs and remedies that were getting her nowhere. Because of her severe symptoms, I insisted she also do a three-day parasite test.

The parasite test came back negative but her CDSA test showed two types of yeast, which were very resistant to natural products. Within ten days of starting on fluconasole, one of the drugs listed that would control both yeast species, she began having a much more normal schedule of two solid bowel movements per day. She continued the drug therapy for an entire month in total, along with natural products to facilitate repair of the bowel. At this point she has gone nine months without a relapse. If she had not cleared up this problem, she very likely would have had to eventually have part of her colon surgically removed.

Her culture and sensitivity tests are shown in the following table. Note how the popular yeast drug, Nystatin, was not the best choice for both yeasts. With the expense of Nystatin, it does not make sense to use it as a trial without this test. I have found Nystatin is not the drug of choice in many of the yeast cultures I have done on my patients.

Comprehensive Digestive Stool Analysis

Great Smokies Diagnostic Laboratory ℠

63 Zillicoa Street
Asheville, North Carolina 28801-1074

Patient:

ID#:   Age: 59   Sex: Female

Collected: 2/15/00   Received: 2/16/00   Completed: 2/22/00

Digestion

	Value	Range
Triglycerides (%)	0.1	0 0.3 2
Chymotrypsin (IU/g)	59.2	0 6.2 41 75
Valerate, iso-Butyrate (umoles/g)	3.4	0 10 30

	Normal	Abnormal	Ref.
Meat Fibers	0		0
Veg. Fibers	1		0-2

Absorption

	Value	Range
LCFAs (%)	1.5	0 1.1 5
Cholesterol (%)	0.4	0 0.3 2
Total fecal fat (%)	1.9	0 1.6 5
Total SCFAs (umoles/g)	46	0 56 156 200

Colonic Environment

Microbiology

Beneficial Bacteria
- Lactobacillus — 3+
- Bifidobacterium — 2+
- Escherichia coli — 4+

Additional Bacteria
- Gamma strep — 2+

Metabolic Markers

	Value	Range
n-Butyrate (umoles/g)	4.9	0 10 30 100
B-Glucuronidase (IU/g)	32	0 300 600
pH	7.5	6 7.2 9

SCFA distribution:
- % Acetate (54-67%) — 73
- % Propionate (16-24%) — 17
- % n-Butyrate (14-23%) — 11
  (0   25   50   75   100)

Immunology

	Value	Range
Fecal sIgA (ug/g)	85	0 44 183 260

Mycology
- Candida albicans — 4+
- Candida parapsilosis — 4+

Microscopic yeast from parasite exam: Few Yeast

Macroscopic

	Optimal	Abnormal	Ref.
Color	BROWN		Brown
Mucus	None		None
Occult blood	Negative		None

Histograms represent idealized data based upon large populations

normal flora   imbalanced flora   possible pathogen

Additional Tests

	Normal	Abnormal	Ref.		Normal	Abnormal	Ref.
Campylobacter specific antigen	Negative		Negative	Enterohemorrhagic Escherichia coli cytotoxin	Negative		Negative

Bacterial Dysbiosis Index

14

0 OPTIMAL 4 SLIGHT 7 MODERATE 11 SEVERE 20

© GSDL • College of American Pathologists #31722-01 • CLIA Lic.#34D0655571 • Medicare Lic. #34-8475 •   g\rp\cdsa\100097

Case #1	Candida albicans			Candida parapsilosis		
	Most Sensitive	Sensitive	Least Sensitive	Most Sensitive	Sensitive	Least Sensitive
Prescriptive Agents						
Fluconazole	<0.5			<0.5		
Itraconazole	<0.5			<0.5		
Ketoconazole	<0.5			<0.5		
Nystatin	<2					10
Natural Substances						
Berberine		160		8		
Caprylic Acid			>500			>500
Garlic		500			500	
Undecylenic			1000		500	
Plant Tannins		8				160
Uva Ursi		160				500

CASE 2

This case involved a forty-four-year-old woman who has suffered from fibromyalgia and chronic fatigue syndrome, since 1986. She had overcome most of her fatigue and muscle aches, but still had persistent memory and concentration problems, as well as chronic vaginal discharge and itching. Her CDSA test showed two problematic organisms, a bacteria, ***Pseudomonas aeruginosa*** (not shown) and a ***Candida*** listed as "Candida species."

Note on her yeast culture and sensitivity test below how the two most popular yeast drugs, Fluconazole (Diflucan) and Nystatin were not the most effective drugs for her yeast problems. Also note with this patient that caprylic acid and garlic were ineffective; both of which are popular natural products used to treat yeast. As with many cases, no natural product was strong enough to effectively treat this woman's yeast condition.

CASE 3

This patient suffered from frequent vaginal yeast infections, fatigue, depression, food and alcohol cravings, PMS and a genital itch during her periods. Her CDSA revealed a bacteria that required treatment and a less common yeast known as ***Rhodotorula*** species, which we affectionately nicknamed "Roto Rooter."

The most fascinating thing about this yeast is there was only one product (Ketoconazole) that would effectively get it under control. She had been given numerous prescriptions of the popular drug, fluconazole (Diflucan), which was shown to be ineffective for this yeast. Itraconazole and Nystatin were also shown to be poor choices.

Berberine, garlic and undecylenic acid showed to be mildly sensitive, indicating they were good choices for follow-up to drug therapy. Caprylic acid, again, proved ineffective.

Case #2	Candida Species		
	Most Sensitive	Sensitive	Least Sensitive
Prescriptive Agents			
Fluconazole			160
Itraconazole	<0.5		
Ketoconazole	<0.5		
Nystatin		10	
Natural Substances			
Berberine			
Caprylic Acid			>500
Garlic			1000
Undecylenic		500	
Plant Tannins		8	
Uva Ursi		160	

Case #3	Rhodotorula Species		
	Most Sensitive	Sensitive	Least Sensitive
Prescriptive Agents			
Fluconazole			160
Itraconazole			>160
Ketoconazole	<0.5		
Nystatin			50
Natural Substances			
Berberine		160	
Caprylic Acid			>500
Garlic		500	
Undecylenic		500	
Plant Tannins			160
Uva Ursi			500

CASE 4

This patient was a forty-five-year-old man who had a veritable zoo of bad germs growing in his GI tract. He suffered from diarrhea for one year, fatigue that was interfering with his ability to work, depression, headaches, memory and concentration problems. He was getting nowhere with the therapies of his GI specialist.

His test showed 1+ *Citrobacter freundii*, a germ famous for causing diarrhea and immune reactions similar to *Salmonella*. *Citrobacter* possesses a toxin similar to some of the more harmful species of *E. Coli.* He also had 4+ *Klebsiella pneumoniae*, which can cause bladder infections, pneumonia, prostatitis and an autoimmune spinal arthritis known as Ankylosing Spondylitis. His most dangerous germ was a 3+ *Staphalococcus aureus,* which is a major cause of food poisoning that can cause abdominal cramps and diarrhea. It has also been implicated in colitis and toxic shock syndrome. Last but not least, our friend, *Candida albicans*, showed up at 4+ (not shown).

Luckily, the three bacteria species could all be treated with the same antibiotic, the herb uva ursi, or a natural herbal product emphasizing plant tannins. This is such a wonderful benefit of the culture and sensitivity test. So many doctors try multiple antibiotics and sometimes never hit the right one for the job. Meanwhile, all of this excessive use of antibiotics exacerbates antibiotic resistance and makes yeast problems even worse.

Between the diarrhea and bad germs sapping his vitality, it is no wonder this man was so exhausted. He continues to make excellent progress since his drug therapies and is rebuilding his intestinal environment with natural therapies.

Case #4	Citrobactor freundii			Klebsiella pneumoniae			Staphylococcus aureus		
	Most Sensitive	Sensitive	Least Sensitive	Most Sensitive	Sensitive	Least Sensitive	Most Sensitive	Sensitive	Least Sensitive
Prescriptive Agents									
Amoxicillin/Clauvuanate				<=8,S					
Ampicillin/Sulbactam							<=4,S		
Carbenicillin	<=16,S								
Cefonicid	<=4,S			<=4,S					
Cephalothin				<=2,S			8,S		
Ciproxfloxacin	<=0.5,S			<=0.5,S			<=0.5,S		
Tetracycline	2,S			2,S			<=1,S		
Trimethoprim/Sulfa	<=10,S			<=10,S			<=10,S		
Clindamycin							<=0.5,S		
Erthromycin							<=0.5,S		
Oxacillin							0.5,S		
Penicillin									>16,R
Vencomycin							<=0.5,S		
Natural Substances									
Berberine			>10000			>10000	>1250		
Oregano		1250			1250			1250	
Plant Tannins	1600			1600			<160		
Uva Ursi	15000			10000			<5000		

CASE 5

This case involves a thirty-seven-year-old woman who was so fatigued she wanted to take a two-hour nap every afternoon. Her primary complaint, however, was that she had been unable to conceive for the past two years. She had previously given birth to two children. A four-month trial with the fertility drug Clomid was unsuccessful and had caused her to have multiple vaginal yeast infections, with severe itching. She also reported that she had severe PMS for the previous two years with cramps, diarrhea and a stomach ache.

This reminded me of a patient I had about ten years ago who was infertile for six years. A fertility specialist finally determined her cervical mucus was killing off her husband's sperm. I explained to her that I believed this meant her mucus contained a flora environment that contained hostile germs. Without even doing this **CDSA** test I put her on some natural products to help kill bad germs. Then I used healthy bacteria to take their place. I also taught her eating habits that would discourage the overgrowth of unhealthy germs. To everyone's delight she became pregnant in five months.

The **CDSA** of Case 5 revealed she had two types of *Klebsiella* germs (not shown) and two types of yeast interfering with her health. She also had absolutely no beneficial bacteria to fight her battles. From her culture and sensitivity tests it was evident that neither of the two popular anti-yeast drugs (fluconazole and nystatin) would have been effective in killing off the *lusitaniae* species. It is also interesting that caprylic acid was helpful this time for both species of yeast. At this point, four months after her therapies, she is not yet pregnant but has much more energy.

Case #5	Candida albicans			Candida lusitaniae		
	Most Sensitive	Sensitive	Least Sensitive	Most Sensitive	Sensitive	Least Sensitive
Prescriptive Agents						
Fluconazole	<0.5				2	
Itraconazole	<0.5			<0.5		
Ketoconazole	<0.5			<0.5		
Nystatin		10			10	
Natural Substances						
Berberine		160			160	
Caprylic Acid	125			250		
Garlic		500			500	
Undecylenic	160				500	
Plant Tannins		8			8	
Uva Ursi		160			160	

Just like bacteria, yeast organisms can have resistance to drugs and natural remedies. What works for one may not for another. While Candida infestations may not be deadly to the average person, they can certainly interfere with our health and vitality. These tests also verify that you cannot assume that every problem with yeast symptoms is ***Candida albicans*** species or even yeast acting alone.

Proper diagnosis from a stool sample is essential to restoring health and vitality. The days of guessing which drug to use should be over. I believe all physicians should use this valuable test to investigate a wide variety of chronic health problems. If you would like to find out more about the **CDSA** test, access the web site for **Great Smokies** lab at **www.gsdl.com** or call them at (800) 522-4762. Both sources can help you find a doctor who does this type of testing. If you are unable to find someone near you, we offer this test in combination with diet, nutrition and lifestyle coaching through our website, **www.vitalitydoctor.com.** However, you would be referred to your family doctor for any drug therapies needed.

CHRONIC SINUSITIS AND YEAST

A recent study by the **Mayo Clinic** found that ninety-three percent of sinus infections were caused by yeast rather than bacteria or viruses. I have met hundreds of patients in my career who have felt compelled to keep going back on antibiotics for their recurrent sinus infections. Some of them could not be convinced that antibiotics were the main reason their infections kept recurring. Yeast imbalances are made worse by antibiotics.

DRUG EFFECTS ON THE COLON

One of the contributing factors to bad germs overgrowing in the intestines is the annihilation of our healthy bacteria by such drugs as antibiotics, cortisone, acid blockers, hormones, chemotherapy, etc. For years, doctors have incorrectly assumed our bacteria return on their own.

In March, 2000, I did a **CDSA** on a twenty-four-year-old male who suffered from irritable bowel syndrome, facial blemishes and rashes, occasional upper respiratory infections, multiple fungal toe nails and athlete's foot. He had not taken any antibiotics in the past five months. Yet his **CDSA** showed he still did not have any measurable levels of beneficial bacteria present in his gut. His intestinal environment was so unhealthy that not even the normal ***E. coli*** species would grow there. This same profile was found in the previous case with infertility. After receiving the drug to treat his fungus, as well as bacteria products to restore his natural bacteria, all of his symptoms resolved, including his toe nail fungus.

The inability for some people to restore their colon flora after drug therapies is very important from a public health standpoint. The intestines provide a whopping sixty percent of the body's immune function. These people are more prone to serious infections since their own "natural army" is wiped out. On a daily basis we ingest various germs via food, beverages or water.

More research needs to be done to determine if people who have become seriously ill or died from food or water parasite outbreaks have had antibiotics prescribed in the past year without having used probiotics to restore their beneficial gut flora. Infants, transplant recipients, HIV and AIDS patients may be especially vulnerable.

As I mentioned previously, eating yogurt after drug therapies is no guarantee your bacterial environment will be restored. Most of the yogurt bacteria are not bred to be strong enough to adhere to your intestines and reproduce. However, there is some evidence to suggest that taking therapeutic types of acidophilus and bifidus along with yogurt will enhance the effects of these bacteria.

N-BUTYRATE AND FIBER

Note the CDSA of Case 1 (page 103) low levels of a metabolic marker known as n-butyrate. This substance is made in our intestines by the fermentation of fiber by our beneficial bacteria. It is the primary source of food to maintain the health of our colon's epithelial cells. If you have a combination of low beneficial bacteria and low n-butyrate, you are at greater risk for developing colon cancer.

An April, 2000 issue of the ***New England Journal of Medicine*** published an article about fiber, derived from two studies, involving thousands of people. It concluded that neither consuming a high-fiber, low-fat diet nor eating extra wheat-bran fiber made a difference in preventing colon cancer.

This is an excellent example of designing a faulty research study around a "Magic Bullet" theory that produces invalid results. Almost no single factor is responsible for an outstanding health benefit. It is usually the synergy of two or more factors.

This study involved people over the age of thirty-five, who each had already exhibited signs of colon dysfunction. All previously had at least one non-cancerous polyp removed from their colons. Fiber alone cannot prevent colon cancer. It requires beneficial bacteria to break it down to produce n-butyrate to heal the colon tissue.

When medical researchers stop asking the wrong questions in their studies, they will start getting the right answers. If the people in this study had been given both fiber and beneficial bacteria they would have had a better chance for their colon function to return to normal, thus preventing subsequent cancers. From the two cases mentioned above, we cannot assume the people in this study had adequate numbers of beneficial bacteria living in their intestines. With the widespread use of chlorinated water and antibiotic therapies, we should assume that the average person does not have adequate beneficial intestinal bacteria.

> "The difference between the impossible and the possible lies in a person's determination."
> — Tommy Lasorda

Day 14

"Sacrifice is giving up something good
for something better."
— Unknown

Whole Grains vs. Flour Products

There is nothing more confusing to consumers than the topic of whole grains. We are told to consume whole grains to prevent heart disease, cancer, obesity and diabetes. But what does "whole" mean? In reality, consuming what you think is a whole grain may actually ***contribute*** to those health problems.

By definition, a whole grain has all three major elements of the anatomy of a grain: bran (outer layer), endosperm (large middle mass) and germ (core). What the food industry calls "whole-grain food" has at least fifty-one percent whole grain by weight. That does not sound very "whole" grain to me.

I prefer the definition of whole grain as "something that would sprout if you soaked it in water." That automatically cuts out anything made from flour. Many flour products, made primarily from refined grains, turn into a pasty substance during digestion and tend to absorb too much water from the bowel. This is a common cause for constipation.

Processing removes bran, which is the fiber that helps prevent cancer, obesity and diabetes. Removing the germ takes out vitamin E. The true whole grains are brown rice, whole-wheat kernels, whole oats, barley (not pearled), buckwheat, quinoa (pronounced keenwa) and millet.

Decreasing flour products is important from a health standpoint because they are similar to refined sugar in their effects on blood sugar and the depletion of nutrients. My patients have seen tremendous benefits in their energy and vitality when they decrease or totally eliminate flour products from their diet.

The book, ***Eat Right For Your Blood Type***, by **Dr. Peter J. D'Adamo**, has some interesting theories about the suitability of various foods, including grains, based on your blood type. I have known several people who have benefited from this information.

Many of my colleagues have remarked that following the advice in **Dr. D'Adamo's** book allowed several of their patients to lose weight after previously being unsuccessful. My advice for losing weight has always included the elimination of flour products and sugar.

OATS AND SPROUTED GRAINS

The oatmeal we commonly think of as "whole" is processed by first soaking it in water and then crushing the kernel. This decreases the cooking time to twenty minutes, while genuine whole oats take an entire hour or more to cook. Some cultures cook oats at low temperatures all night, for example in a crock-pot.

Be aware that many sprouted wheat breads often contain only small amounts of sprouted wheat and are primarily flour-based breads. The exception is Essene and Ezekiel breads, which are one hundred percent sprouted wheat breads. They are often found in health food store refrigerators or freezers. They are a live food, with many beneficial enzymes intact. The gluten lectin, which is so troubling to many people's digestive tract, is destroyed in the sprouting process.

If you are going to make your own breads from flour, you should consider flour products to be as perishable as milk and grind your flours from whole grains immediately before baking. Many stores carry flour-grinding machines. A stone-grinding machine is best.

When my son was an infant, I used to make all his whole grain cereals by grinding them with a small coffee grinder. The most common grains I used were brown rice, millet and buckwheat. I used to fortify the cereals with iron by using a liver food concentrate called **Ferrofood®** from **Standard Process Labs**. There is only ten mg. of iron per capsule so it was easy to take a small amount of iron for the batch of cereal I was making. The RDA for iron in children, one-ten years of age, is ten mg.

TODAY'S ACTIVITY

Check out your food and activity diary. Circle the number of servings of flour products you consume in one day: bread, pasta, bagels, pancakes, waffles, English muffins, breakfast cereal, pastry, donuts, toaster items, cookies, gravy, soups with macaroni, noodles or flour thickeners, etc. Start eliminating flour products for at least four to five day periods. In the coming weeks, start to notice your energy levels on the days (or day after) you consume flour products.

COOKING WITH WHOLE GRAIN

The primary ways to cook whole grains include boiling, pressure-cooking and roasting the grain first in a dry skillet before boiling. The latter method creates a lighter texture and nutty flavor. I recommend you start with brown rice and millet. Brown rice is available in short grain, which is best for most purposes. Long grain rice works quite well in soups.

Brown basmati and the various varieties by **Lundberg Farms**, found in health food stores, each have distinctive flavors you may prefer. Millet is basically the same as birdseed, but is a wonderful little grain that cooks up quicker than rice and can be prepared in a variety of ways.

Experiment with less commonly used grains such as barley, quinoa, buckwheat and whole oats. Barley and oats have high gluten like wheat, so avoid if you are sensitive. Brown rice, barley and whole oats take forty-five to sixty minutes cooking time and millet, quinoa, and buckwheat take twenty to thrity minutes to cook.

Cooking Instructions

1) In general, cook grains with three parts water to one part grain. You can substitute soymilk, rice milk or nut milk as part of the liquid, if you would like a more creamy breakfast grain. You can also add a dash of cinnamon and some raisins for flavor.

2) Start boiling the liquid while you rinse the grain in a metal strainer. Millet and quinoa are very tiny and need a strainer with a tight mesh. I usually put the strainer on top of a quart liquid container and let the water fill up around the grain to wash it thoroughly. I change the water three times to clean the grain well.

3) Add the rinsed grain to boiling water and then add sea salt after it begins to boil again. Cover and reduce the heat to low and cook until the water is absorbed. Electric and high altitude cooking will take longer than gas. Grains with a long cooking time can be started in the morning and then finished when you get home.

Suggestions

Experiment with adding vegetables and squashes to grains to enhance the flavor. Quinoa definitely tastes better with vegetables cooked into it. Millet has some of the most interesting effects from vegetables. When you cook it with cauliflower it takes on the flavor of mashed potatoes. When you add butternut squash and onions it tastes very sweet.

You may want to cook two or more grains together for a more interesting flavor. Rice and barley make a good combination. Try adding sliced cabbage and carrots, peas and corn or winter squash that has been peeled and cut. Be adventurous! Try grains and vegetables you have not had before. Check out cookbooks that feature less reliance on flour and refined sugar. Our web site, **www.vitalitydoctor.com** features *The Guilt-Free Indulgence Cookbook*, written by my Health Coach® mentor, **Dr. Mark Percival,** and his wife, **Cheri**. It is an excellent source for obtaining healthy and tasty recipes.

ORIENTAL WISDOM

Another reason to consider eating a greater variety of grains, other than only wheat, is that according to Oriental medicine, each grain nourishes different organs. If you only eat one type of grain, you nourish only certain organs and your other organs may become weak. The nourished organs also may develop excessive energy.

Oriental medicine acknowledges that wheat nourishes the liver and gall bladder, rice nourishes the lungs and large intestine, rye nourishes the spleen and pancreas, and millet nourishes the heart and small intestine. The kidney and bladder are nourished by beans, especially kidney beans and a small red bean known as aduki.

In a short time, you will notice eating cooked whole grains will give you more even, sustained energy than flour products. They are a whole, complete food and are metabolized much more slowly. This will lead to greater insulin balance and curb blood sugar fluctuations. Stabilization of blood sugar allows you to burn fat for energy and maintain a more normal weight.

> "One cannot think well, love well, sleep well,
> if one has not dined well."
> — Virginia Woolf

Day 15

"Discipline is the bridge between goals
and accomplishments."

— Jim Rohn

MOOve Away from Dairy

Dairy foods come from lactating cows, goats and sheep, and are products such as milk, butter, cheese, yogurt and cream. Because eggs are sold in the grocery store's dairy department, some people mistakenly associate eggs as a dairy food. I mention this because when I ask people to decrease their dairy intake, some get confused and wonder if they can still eat eggs.

Milk is the perfect food for newborns. Cow's milk is the perfect food for calves. Cow's milk is designed to help a calf double its weight in the first six weeks of life. Cow's milk and goat's milk have almost three times the amount of protein as human milk, but only half the carbohydrates. These differences are undoubtedly a factor in the ever-increasing height and weight of Americans. This is consistent with the increased obesity in children who are bottle-fed with cow's milk formula compared to those who are breast-fed.

Only a minority of people in the world continue to consume milk past weaning. These are mostly countries with a predominant Caucasian population. Many countries consume fewer dairy products than the U.S. and their dairy products have less processing, drugs and additives. Dairy cattle in the U.S. are given hormones, tranquilizers and antibiotics. Our milk products are homogenized, irradiated, preserved, colored and supplemented with vitamins.

Excessive consumption of dairy products is believed to contribute to a variety of health problems. Most people believe fat content is the only problem with dairy products, and they consume low fat and skim varieties. However, the lactose (milk sugar) and casein (milk protein) seem to cause significant problems as well.

The milk industry would have us believe we cannot possibly get enough calcium in our diets without dairy foods. My question to people who have this concern is, "When was the last time you had a grilled cheese sandwich in a Chinese restaurant?" Asians and Africans get along fine without dairy foods in their diets. In fact, the majority of people in these cultures, are lactose intolerant and become sick from dairy products.

Many people suffer from undiagnosed lactose intolerance. Nursing infants can digest lactose in human milk because they receive the lactase enzyme directly from the mother. By age five, a child's ability to synthesize lactase begins to decrease. This is just in time for the school lunch program where many children are forced to drink milk.

By adulthood, about seventy percent of the world's population has negligible production of lactase, resulting in lactose intolerance. The symptoms of lactose intolerance include abdominal cramps, gas, nausea, bloating and diarrhea. Despite this, people with these symptoms are sometimes told by their doctors they do not have lactose intolerance, even when avoidance of dairy brings relief.

LACTOSE INTOLERANCE IN ETHNIC POPULATIONS

*From *Clinical Nutrition: A Functional Approach.*, Dr. Jeffrey Bland
Copyright © 1999 by the **Institute For Functional Medicine™, Inc.**

Ethnic Group	% Lactose intolerant
African Blacks	97-100
Orientals	90-100
North American Blacks	70-75
Mexicans	70-80
Mediterraneans	60-90
Jewish Descent	60-80
Middle Europeans	10-20
North American Caucasians	7-15
Northern Europeans	1-5

Lactase supplementation will help some people who are unable to digest lactose. It is most effective when added directly to liquid milk. Lactase will not help if a person's dairy sensitivity is to casein. Because casein protein is a common reactive substance associated with immune-based food allergies, dairy often needs to be eliminated in people with chronic allergies. Anyone with hay fever, asthma, sinusitis or skin conditions such as acne, eczema or psoriasis should avoid dairy for fourteen to thirty days to see how it impacts their condition. I frequently recommend to the majority of my patients they either drastically reduce their intake for awhile or avoid dairy products altogether.

Many infants and children are misdiagnosed with colds and sinus problems that develop into ear infections simply because they cannot digest cow's milk. They develop tremendous amounts of congestion that clog the ear tubes, which drain into the throat. Some ear, nose and throat surgeons are significantly decreasing the need for ear tube surgeries by first requesting the child stop consuming dairy. This is also the case for sinus surgeries in adults.

Eliminating dairy from the diet can be an emotionally charged decision in America. Parents who take this approach toward improving their children's health are often met with opposition from their doctors, school and daycare providers, and family members. Parents are often made to feel that avoiding dairy can be detrimental to their child's health, when in fact, the opposite may be true. In my practice I have seen both adults and children who suffered fewer infections and improved their levels of memory and concentration by eliminating dairy foods. Tantrums and aggressive behavior in children may also be improved by avoiding dairy.

COMMON SOURCES OF LACTOSE
*From *Clinical Nutrition: A Functional Approach.*, Dr. Jeffrey Bland
Copyright © 1999 by the **Institute For Functional Medicine™, Inc.**

Obvious Sources

- All cheeses
- Butter, many margarines
- Goat's milk
- Half-and-half cream
- Ice cream and sherbet
- Milk (whole, skim, dry powered, evaporated)
- Yogurt

"Hidden" Sources

- Artificial sweeteners
- Breads, biscuits, crackers, and donuts made with milk
- Breading on fried foods
- Breakfast and baby cereals containing milk solids
- Buttered or creamed foods like soups and vegetables
- Cake and pudding mixes, many frostings
- Candies made with milk chocolate
- Cookies made with milk
- Hotdogs, luncheon meats, sausage, hash, processed and canned meats
- Mayonnaise and salad dressings made with milk
- Nondairy creamers (except for Coffee Rich®)
- Pancakes, waffles, toaster tarts
- Pizza
- Weight-reduction formulas
- Many prescription drugs, including allergy drugs, birth control pills, thyroid medication, and medications for gastrointestinal disorders (Reglan and Xanax)
- Many types of vitamins
  *Plus any food labeled as containing whey, casein, caseinate, sodium caseinate, and lactose

PERSONAL STORY

Substituting soy or rice milk for cow's milk is becoming much more common. My son has never used cow's milk as a beverage. He has had some cheese and yogurt but always drank soymilk when he was young. That, combined with the fact that he nursed until two years of age allowed him to get through his childhood without needing a single round of antibiotics. He is now fifteen and has strong bones, good teeth and no problems with his dental occlusion.

This is a sharp contrast to my "dairy rich" childhood. I was the "first to get sick and the last to get well." I had so many sore throats and ear infections that my tonsils were removed at age seven. My problems with frequent infections did not stop until age twenty-two when I changed my diet. I have now gone twenty-five years without needing antibiotics for infections. Eating only small amounts of dairy once or twice a week also has allowed my sore throats, sinus problems and hay fever to be totally eliminated.

There are many more things that damage teeth and bones than a lack of calcium. We have known for years that eating candy will damage teeth, even though they are the hardest substances in our bodies. If sugars can demineralize teeth, they can certainly contribute to bone loss. High phosphorus intake, such as from soda pop and excessive meat consumption, will contribute greatly to osteoporosis.

Soda pop also contains caffeine and ten teaspoons of sugar per can, both of which are severely damaging to the health of young people. Children start this habit young with fast food meals. One popular fast food chain reports forty percent of its total business comes from children's meals. Even though it feels wasteful to request water instead of the soft drink that comes with the meal, it is more detrimental to instill a habit in children that soda is an acceptable beverage for meals.

By the time children become teenagers they are conditioned to believe that soda is a "normal" part of their diet and their consumption becomes far too frequent. Many young people are starting their day with a caffeine soda drink, much like the older generations skip breakfast and just drink coffee. These are both very destructive health habits that need to stop. Parents should be setting an example for their children by serving a proper breakfast.

TODAY'S ACTIVITY

Note on your Food and Activity diaries how many dairy products you are consuming. If you are consuming something containing dairy on a daily basis, you could benefit from a trial abstinence. Even if you did not choose to decrease your dairy intake on Day 8, give it a short trial. Eliminate all dairy products for five days and then add them back. This should tell you by the following day if you have some symptoms related to dairy.

Sometimes when people first stop using dairy, their nose and sinuses start to clear and you may notice a few days or weeks of excessive discharge. This has been so dramatic in some of my clients that they mistakenly thought they had a cold. If this happens to you, stay away from dairy until this entire process is over. It is also very wise to abstain from dairy whenever you have a nose, throat or lung infection.

Note whether you wake up feeling more congested after you add dairy back into your diet. You may find, like me, that it is not worth eating dairy products more than once per week.

In addition to many soy milks offering calcium fortification, nuts, beans and green leafy vegetables are good natural sources of calcium. The following table lists alternative sources of calcium. It does not include sea vegetables, which were mentioned in **Day 10-Green Inside is Clean Inside**.

NONDAIRY HIGH-CALCIUM FOODS

From *Clinical Nutrition: A Functional Appraoch*, Dr. Jeffrey Bland
© 1999 Institute for Functional Medicine ™, Inc.

Approximate milligrams (mg) calcium content per 8 oz (1 cup)

Vegetables
330	Bok choy, cooked
320	Bean sprouts
250	Spinach, cooked
260	Collard greens, cooked
450	Mustard greens, cooked
450	Turnip greens, cooked

Nuts
660	Almonds
600	Chestnuts
450	Filberts
280	Walnuts
900	Sesame seeds
260	Sunflower seeds

Beans
340	Garbanzo beans, cooked
450	Soybeans, cooked
400	Tofu

Nut Butters
270	Almond
195	Filbert
426	Sesame
120	Sunflower
40	Peanut

Fish
300	Raw oysters
130	Shrimp
490	Salmon with bones
680	Mackerel, canned with bones
1000	Sardines, canned with bones

Grains
300	Tapioca
20	Brown rice, cooked
80	Quinoa, cooked
50	Corn meal, whole grain
40	Rye flour, dark
20	Rye flour, light

Nut Milks
400	Sesame butter (100 gm) + 2 Tbsp molasses + water
300	Almond (100 gm) + honey + water
200	Filbert + maple syrup + water

"Your goals are the road maps that guide you and show you what is possible for your life."
— Les Brown

3 DAY FOOD & ACTIVITY DIARY

	Date:	Date:	Date:
Morning Meal Time:			
Snack			
Noon Meal Time:			
Snack			
Evening Meal Time:			
Snack			
Symptoms (Physical & Emotional)			
Exercise Type & Duration			

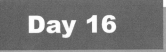
Day 16

Water & Dehydration

Water is the most essential element for survival and functioning. In the United States, we are privileged to have some of the safest drinking water in the world. This factor alone has a lot to do with our longevity. Many countries have inadequate or unclean water for bathing and drinking, which causes rampant parasite diseases. Despite nearly thirty years of federal cleanup efforts, the U.S. still has forty percent of its rivers, lakes, streams and coastal waters that are too polluted for people to fish or swim in.

Water is used throughout our bodies for cellular functions, digestion and elimination. The following chart details some important roles of water.

FUNCTIONS OF WATER
• The brain is seventy-five percent water. Moderate dehydration can cause headaches and dizziness.   • Water distributes nutrients, oxygen, electrolytes, hormones and other chemical messengers throughout the body.   • Water is required for expiration.   • Water moistens oxygen for breathing.   • Water is involved in energy production and the regulation of body temperature.   • Blood is ninety-two percent water.   • Water protects and cushions vital organs and joints. It is an important structural component of skin, cartilage and other tissues.   • Water helps the body absorb nutrients and remove wastes.   • Bones are twenty-two percent water. Muscles are seventy-five percent water.

The importance of water in regulating body temperature cannot be overemphasized. Strenuous outdoor activity requires plenty of water, not soft drinks, to prevent heat stroke. For activities less than two hours long, you will only require water for replacement. For longer periods of exertion, you should choose a fluid replacement product with a low sugar content.

When fighting a fever, you also need ample amounts of water. The nervous system functions very poorly in a state of dehydration, which can severely hinder the healing process. If the brain becomes overheated quickly, it can result in convulsions. Restoring fluids can produce rapid improvement.

PERSONAL STORY

When my son was eighteen months old, I was having difficulty getting his fever down because I could not get him to drink anything. He was absolutely miserable and lethargic. Finally, I recalled hearing that a cool water enema (the approximate temperature of tap water in the summer) would bring down a fever. As much as I did not relish the idea of doing this to my poor child, I will never forget the results. I put him in the bathtub because I was afraid he would immediately expel the water. Within one minute of inserting a small amount of water he became happy and energetic. I could not believe the difference in his well-being. He never did have diarrhea. About three hours later he had a normal bowel movement. It was a dramatic lesson in the healing power of water.

Despite our plentiful supply, many Americans are not getting adequate amounts of water in their daily diet. A recent survey showed that nearly ten percent said they drink no water at all, and twenty-eight percent drink only two servings of water per day. Drinking six to eight eight-ounce glasses of water per day is the suggested guideline to replace what we lose. It is estimated we lose ten to twelve cups of water daily through digestion, urination, sweat and breathing.

Alcohol and caffeine from sodas, coffee and tea are big culprits for causing a diuretic effect, which creates dehydration. Any beverage (including water) that is ice cold will lead to excessive urination. When urinating, you are not only passing pure water from your kidneys, but numerous minerals as well. Therefore, I caution people against using nutrient-depleting drinks, such as coffee and soda, in their daily diet.

CANCER PREVENTION

Cancer prevention is another reason to drink more water. Research indicates a high intake of fluids dilutes the concentration of cancer-causing agents in urine; reducing the bladder's exposure to toxins. **Harvard** researchers watched a group of 47,909 men, ages forty to seventy-five, over a ten-year period. They found that drinking six or more eight-ounce cups of water each day resulted in a fifty-one percent reduction in the risk of bladder cancer. This is the *fourth leading type of cancer* in men, so they must not be drinking enough water.

A study published in the *Journal of the American Dietetic Association* suggested that women who drank at least five glasses of water a day had a forty-five percent lower risk of colon cancer. Other studies have suggested that increasing fluid intake can also lower the risk of prostate, kidney and breast cancer.

IS DEHYDRATION AFFECTING YOUR HEALTH?

Exercise, driving and flying all greatly increase the need for water. If you wait until you are thirsty, you are already dehydrated. A general guideline is to drink twelve ounces of water for every thirty minutes of exercise, or every hour you are in a plane or car.

One way to look for dehydration, if you have not recently consumed B vitamins, is to observe the color of your urine. Amber or dark yellow urine is the classic sign of dehydration. The riboflavin in B vitamins will also color your urine bright yellow, but this is no cause for concern.

TODAY'S ACTIVITY

Note the following symptoms of dehydration. Check off those symptoms you have at least once every three days and then come back to this list a week after you have made a diligent effort to drink six to eight glasses per day. You will discover how many of these symptoms were related to the simple habit of drinking more water throughout the day.

Present Symptoms

One Week Later

❑ yellow or dark urine ___

❑ mid-day grogginess ___

❑ dry lips and tongue ___

❑ apathy and lack of energy ___

❑ muscle cramping ___

❑ concentration loss ___

❑ headache ___

❑ indigestion ___

❑ constipation ___

❑ red, flushed face ___

❑ sunken eyes ___

HOW SAFE IS YOUR WATER?

Bottled waters have become very popular because people are concerned about germs and pollutants in our drinking water. Even though the U.S. enjoys some of the best quality drinking water in the world, a 1996 study by the nonprofit **Natural Resources Council (NRDC)** and the nonprofit research organization, **Environmental Working Group,** found water treatment is far from perfect.

Using data from the **Environmental Protection Agency**, they reported more than forty-five million Americans, during 1994 and 1995, were drinking tap water polluted with fecal matter, parasites, radiation, disease-causing microbes, pesticides, toxic chemicals and lead.

Since 1974, the number of contaminants regulated by the **Safe Drinking Water Act** has grown from thirteen to ninety, ranging from dioxin, an industrial and agricultural byproduct, to naturally occurring toxins like radon.

In 1995, the **Centers for Disease Control** and the **Environmental Protection Agency** concluded that an estimated 940,000 Americans per year were getting sick from contaminated tap water. As many as one-third of gastrointestinal illnesses, blamed on the flu, were actually caused by drinking water. Even more surprising, tap water kills about nine hundred people each year, often when their immune systems are already compromised. This is an important reason why infant formula should *always* be mixed with good quality filtered water.

The Milwaukee *Cryptosporidum* outbreak in April, 1993, occurred even though their water treatment facility was meeting federal safety standards at the time. This devastating epidemic caused *400,000* people to suffer flu-like symptoms, and 104 to die. *Cryptosporidium* is a very tiny organism that is resistant to chlorine. This makes it difficult to filter out or disinfect in water.

Even clean tap water contains low levels of contaminants. Contamination levels are averaged from several months up to a year. Therefore, a particularly heavy couple of days, where rains or floods deluge a water system with increased agricultural and lawn runoff, might not sound any alarms.

RAIN CLOUD CONTAMINATION

Stephen Muller, a chemist at the **Swiss General Institute for Environmental Science and Technology**, has reported that much of today's rainwater is contaminated with crop pesticides. Common pesticides such as atrazine, alachlor and others evaporate after being applied to crop fields and then combine with the water vapor in clouds. These pesticides are so concentrated in rain clouds soon after application, that the subsequent rain would be illegal to use as drinking water.

In Europe, laws require that drinking water contain no more than one hundred nanograms of pesticides per liter of water. In their tests of rain samples from forty-one different storms, nine contained more than one hundred nanograms of atrazine per liter, one had nine hundred nanograms and one had four thousand nanograms per liter.

WATER TREATMENT

Several water treatment changes have occurred since the Milwaukee *Cryptosporidium* outbreak, but it will never be one hundred percent safe. Chlorination may be necessary from a public health standpoint but it is not without risks. A study published in the ***American Journal of Public Health*** 1997;87:1168-1176, demonstrated a "clear dose-response relation" between the chloroform levels (a water chlorination by-product) and colon cancer (including all cancers) in post-menapausal women in Iowa. The following graph shows a seventy-two percent increase in colon cancer for Iowa women, who drank chlorinated city water, compared to water from ground water sources. All cancers increased by thirty percent.

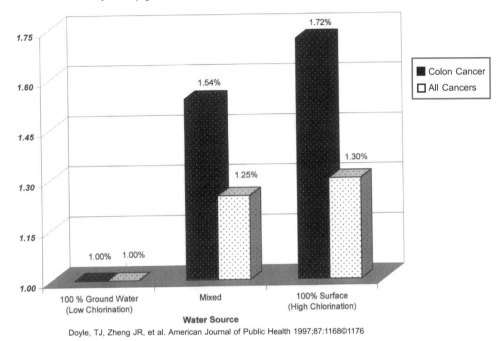

Doyle, TJ, Zheng JR, et al. American Journal of Public Health 1997;87:1168©1176

In addition to the risk of cancer, the colon bacterial environment is very susceptible to death from chlorine. This is why you should consider taking probiotic bacteria such as ***acidophilus*** and ***bifidus*** every week if you regularly consume unfiltered, chlorinated water.

DRINKING WATER PURIFICATION

There are a variety of water purifying methods, such as carbon filtration, ozonation, ultraviolet light exposure and photo-oxidation. Some water purifiers combine two or more of these methods. Reverse osmosis and distillation are two other methods of water treatment that take a little more time than a faucet filter. Shower filtration attachments are also available.

Using a filtered pitcher or water bottle, such as those by **Brita®,** is a very inexpensive method for filtering out chlorine. Be sure to change the filters regularly. While filters are great for improving taste and decreasing chlorine, there are varying degrees of success at removing heavy metals, parasites, pesticides and herbicides. Filters also lose their effectiveness over time.

Distillation is the only method that removes the water from the contaminants, rather than the contaminants from the water. A distiller turns water into steam, which passes through a stainless steel coil. It then passes through a filter, which absorbs volatile organic compounds. After that stage, it is collected and stored.

A good quality distillation system will remove virtually every kind of bacteria, virus, parasite, and pathogen. It will also separate the water from pesticides, herbicides, organic and inorganic chemicals, heavy metals and even radioactive contaminants. A good one-gallon distillation unit can be obtained for less than $500 and uses only pennies of electricity per gallon.

HOME FILTRATION

You may want to consider having a whole-house filtration unit installed. About sixty-four to ninety-one percent of exposure to waterborne contaminants is known to occur through absorption by the skin. This can occur from both bathing and washing clothes.

Having worked as a dental hygienist for five years in the 1970's, I was well aware of the ongoing public relations campaign to convince the public that fluoridated water was completely safe. According to **George Glasser**, in the September, 2000 issue of *The Ecologist* (**www.theecologist.org**), the fluoride they are putting in your water may not be the same fluoride used in safety studies.

One dentist did research at his local water department and found they were using hexafluorosilicic acid, an inexpensive toxic waste product from phosphate fertilizer pollution scrubbers. This product contains other toxic substances such as arsenic, beryllium, mercury, lead and many more. The water department manager explained it would be "too expensive to use a good grade of fluoride."

Because of the many issues regarding chemicals and heavy metals in our water, I personally believe you should consider using a whole-house filter plus a water distillation device for your drinking water.

BOTTLED WATERS

A February, 1999 report, by the **Natural Resources Defense Council**, found bottled water is not necessarily cleaner or safer than most tap water. Some twenty percent of bottled waters come from ordinary tap water. The **FDA** requires the label on these bottles indicate "from a community water system" or "from a municipal source" on the label.

To find out which brands of bottled water are **NSF** Certified and comply with **FDA** regulations, visit **www.nsf.org**. **NSF International** also evaluates and sets standards for water filters. They discuss how the various types meet your needs.

Check Your Water Supply

To find out how well your water supply is adhering to **EPA** guidelines you can obtain a **Consumer Confidence Report (CCR)** from your local water supplier or find it online at **www.epa.gov/safewater/ dwinfo.htm.** You may also call the **EPA's Safe Drinking Water Hotline**, (800) 426-4791.

What Are We Bathing In?

In addition to being concerned with our drinking water, we also have to consider the water we swim and bathe in. Radon in tap water, causes lung cancer because it is released as a gas during showers. Triathletes and swimmers have come down with a variety of illnesses from pools, hot tubs, lakes, rivers and ocean beaches.

The following chart shows a variety of germs, found in swimming pools and spas, which can cause a variety of low-grade infections. To prevent more serious contamination, never swim in stagnant or polluted water. Take "no swimming" signs seriously. Avoid swallowing water and try to keep your head above water. Wear ear and nose plugs, goggles or masks.

TYPES OF ILLNESSES RELATED TO POOLS AND SPAS
Colorado State University Environmental Quality Laboratory, Reprinted with permission

Organism	Illness	Symptom
Pseudomonas aeruginosa	Ear Infections	Ear aches, inflamed ears, swollen mucous membranes
Strapylococcus or Pseudomonas	Skin Rash (Dermatitis)	Red pimple-like rashes of the skin, especially around the hair follicles; itching, sore armpits
Mycobacteria	Granulomas (small legions on the skin)	Lesions growing into smaller ulcerated sores
Trichophyton rubrum or Epidermophyton floccosum	Athletes Foot	Itching, scaling, cracking, blistering of feet, especially between toes
Streptococcus or Adenovirus	Pink Eye/Conjunctivitis	Irritation and redness in the eyes, sometimes a slight fever
Bacteria (Shigella, Salmonella), Protozoa (Giardia Cryptosporidium), other bacteria or viruses	Gastroenteritis	Diarrhea, vomiting, possible fever, cramps, fatigue
Bacteria (Pseudomonas, Legionella) Virus (rhinovirus, adenovirus)	Respiratory Illness	Pneumonia, flu-like symptoms, sinus problems, sore throat, cough

Pure water needs to become your favorite beverage. It is imperative to our health that we make a conscious effort to drink plenty of pure water daily. Water purification is a must so our families can receive less exposure to toxins. Even if your water "tastes fine," we still need to take extra steps to remove the chlorine and other chemicals.

We need to make every effort to protect our lakes, rivers and oceans from pollution. With our burgeoning world population, water is going to become more precious than gold.

> "The first wealth is health."
> — Ralph Waldo Emerson

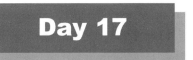

"The higher your energy level, the more efficient your body. The more efficient your body, the better you feel and the more you will use your talent to produce outstanding results."

— Anthony Robbins

Eat Your Veggies!

In our instant-food society, fresh vegetables are often forgotten as being a necessary part of our diets. Five of the six top causes of death in America are diet-related. Yet, more than eighty percent of us do not eat enough fruit and vegetables. This is one of the major contributing factors for the increases in obesity, diabetes and colon cancers. The most recent recommendation is to consume five to eight servings of fruits and vegetables daily.

Colon cancer is striking people at a very young age. Baseball player, **Darryl Strawberry,** has had it twice by age thirty-eight. Today show host, **Katie Couric's** husband died of colon cancer at age forty-two. A few years ago, I had a patient whose husband died of colon and liver cancer at age thirty-three. He was not fond of vegetables.

I have observed many parents who allow their children to shun all vegetables, except for french fries. Indeed, a study published in the October 1, 1998 journal *Cancer*, found that twenty-five percent of all vegetables consumed by Americans were french fries. In addition, I have frequently observed from my clients' diet charts that many people eat only fruits. Some eat a single vegetable but it is often the same vegetable every time.

The goal of my health recommendations frequently involves decreasing sweets, balancing blood sugar and decreasing the food supply to harmful germs and yeast that live in the gut. In order to accomplish this, I must stress that all simple sugars be decreased in the diet, including fruits. Many people who have yeast problems are eating three to five servings of fruit per day. In order to effectively get yeast and other bad germs under control, most people need to decrease fruit to *one* serving per day or less.

This means that of the minimum five servings of fruits and vegetables needed per day, four should be vegetables. This is why I am primarily stressing vegetables in this chapter. Although those who are not suffering from an overgrowth of bad germs in their gut may be able to handle more fruit per day, I do not recommend anyone eat more fruits than vegetables on a regular basis. Even the government guidelines stress two to three fruit servings and three to five vegetable servings per day.

On *Day 10,* I emphasized the importance of green foods. Green is certainly the most predominant color of the plant kingdom, which would indicate that we need a lot of it. But let's not forget the many other colors available from plant foods. In the past decade, nutrition research has discovered incredible healing compounds in every color of fruits and vegetables. There are many compounds yet to be discovered, which are not available in supplement form. We need a wide variety of foods to provide the proper balance of antioxidants.

These compounds in plant foods are called phytonutrients. Plants have had to evolve this type of antioxidant protection to combat the oxidizing effects of ultraviolet radiation from the sun. Phytonutrients are found at their highest levels when a fruit or vegetable has been allowed to ripen fully before harvest. This is why it is extremely important to eat the majority of your fruits and vegetables from local growers. The following table lists the numerous phytonutrients common to each color of food.

PHYTONUTRIENTS COMMONLY FOUND IN FOOD SOURCES		
COLOR	**FOOD SOURCE**	**PHYTONUTRIENT**
Green	Broccoli Cabbage Okra Green Leafy Veggies Beans Spinach	Chlorophyll Carotenoids Sulforaphane Thiocyanates
Orange-Red	Apricots Cantaloupe Carrots Mangos Peppers Pumpkin Tomatoes Squash Yams Watermelon	Carotenes: Lycopene Lutein Zeaxanthin
Purple-Red	All Berries Grapes Red Wine	Anthocyanins Ellagic Acid Reversatrol Quercetin
Yellow	Lemons Other Citrus	Limonene
White	Apples Garlic Onion Family	Allium Allyl Sulfide Quercetin
Cream	Cauliflower Potatoes	Anthoxanthins
Brown	Dried Beans Peanuts Soy	Isoflavones Genestein Daidzein Saponins

It is interesting to note how many people still consume canned vegetables as their primary source of vegetables. With all the variety we have in our grocery stores and summer farmer's markets, this is difficult to fathom. Canned vegetables were a necessity in the days before refrigeration and modern grocery stores. They should be used rarely in this day and age. It is well documented that canned vegetables contain the least amount of nutrients when compared to fresh or frozen.

ACID AND ALKALINE BALANCE

One of the major reasons fruits and vegetables are so important to our daily diet is the issue of acid and alkaline balance. Our cells are slightly alkaline, with a pH of 7.3 to 7.4. Even our blood is slightly alkaline. Most fruits and vegetables break down to an alkaline ash. It is this alkalinity that balances all of the other components of our diets that are acid. Meats, sugar, flours, dairy, soft drinks and coffee are all very acidic to the body.

I test the pH of the saliva on all of my patients to ensure they are getting enough alkaline products in their diets. Ideal salivary pH is around 6.8. People with the most severe health problems nearly always have a low pH. My pH paper only goes as low as 5.0 and there are many people with this reading. Their true pH could be even worse.

I have seen some people whose pH was so low, they were starting to have rampant tooth decay. This is why acidic products like coffee, sugar and refined flours are incompatible with recovering from disease. They create an unfavorable acid environment that makes it difficult for our cells to function properly and be repaired. It would be nearly impossible to eat enough vegetables to overcome the acidity of daily, excessive intakes of acidic foods and beverages.

TODAY'S ACTIVITY

Make a big salad or soup, enough for two to three days. Use at least two vegetables you have not consumed in at least a month. Try to use at least five or six vegetables. This is a great way to get your entire day's total of vegetables in one meal!

If you have chosen to make a salad, try to use vegetables with a variety of colors such as yellow squash, carrots, red pepper, purple cabbage or jicama (white). Choose salad dressings with no sugar, and that have natural ingredients, like vinegar and extra virgin olive oil.

If you have chosen to make a soup, by all means include a source of protein such as meat, beans or tofu. I usually start all soups by sautéing onions in olive oil. Then I add water or stock and start throwing everything else in. Experiment with hearty vegetables like hard winter squashes (butternut, delicata, hokaido, etc.). Try cabbage, leeks, carrots, celery, garlic, ginger and the sea vegetable wakame. You can also use green onions for soup by cutting the white parts into the soup early and chopping the green tops as a garnish just before serving.

Another way to eat plenty of vegetables is to make stir-fry meals. Again, I usually start with onions and then add about four different vegetables. If I am adding meat, I usually add it last. When using tofu as the protein, I dip slices in soy sauce and fry it both sides with no oil in a separate skillet.

The many nutrients in fruits and vegetables protect our bodies through their antioxidant and detoxifying effects. Just as "green inside is clean inside," we need a colorful diet with plenty of variety to protect our organs. Make a concerted effort to increase your vegetable intake and choose fruits instead of sweets and snacks.

The following are some of the beneficial effects recently discovered pertaining to fruits and vegetables.

MANY FRUITS, VEGETABLES AND HERBS ARE BECOMING FAMOUS FOR THEIR DISEASE-PROTECTING QUALITIES:

- **Tomatoes** are a major source of lycopene, which reduces the risk of cancer of the prostate, lung and stomach by forty percent. It also increases cancer survival.

- **Red grapes**, including juice and wine have four times more antioxidant activity than orange or tomato juice.

- **Blueberries** are rich in antioxidants that can slow aging in animals and can both block and reverse failing memory.

- **Garlic** is a powerful antioxidant that can prevent cancer, heart disease and slow the aging process.

- **Spinach** is rich in folic acid, which helps fight cancer, heart disease and mental disorders. Folic acid protects aging brains from degeneration and may help prevent Alzheimer's according to research at the **University of Kentucky**.

- **Broccoli** has been shown to prevent fatal heart disease in a 1999, **University of Minnesota** study.

- **Broccoli and cabbage** consumption causes fifty percent less bladder cancer according to a 1999 **Harvard** study.

- **Cruciferous vegetables** (broccoli, cabbage, kale, cauliflower and Brussels sprouts) have been shown to be very effective at helping liver detoxification, and reducing stomach and colon cancer.

- **Apples and apple juice** contain antioxidants that help prevent clogged arteries, according to tests at the **University of California-Davis Medical Center**.

- **Leafy greens, like spinach, collards, parsley and kale**, are rich in the carotenoids, lutein and zeaxanthin, which may prevent macular degeneration of the eye.

- **Green tea** may prevent cancer and also block decay-causing bacteria from adhering to the teeth.

HEALTH BENEFITS FROM HIGH ORAC FOODS

The **U.S. Department of Agriculture (USDA)**, recently tested a wide variety of foods for what they call their ORAC (Oxygen Radical Absorbance Capacity). This is a measure of the antioxidant potential of a food to neutralize free radicals. The higher the ORAC value of a food, the more beneficial it is to your health.

ORAC VALUES OF FRUITS AND VEGETABLES
(PER 100 GRAMS, OR 3.5 OUNCES)

Fruits		Vegetables	
Prunes	5,770	Kale	1,770
Raisins	2,830	Spinach, raw	1,260
Blueberries	2,400	Brussels sprouts	980
Blackberries	2,036	Alfalfa sprouts	930
Cranberries	1,750	Spinach, steamed	909
Strawberries	1,540	Broccoli florets	890
Raspberries	1,220	Beets	841
Plums	949	Red bell pepper	713
Oranges	750	Onion	450
Grapes, red	739	Corn	400
Cherries	670	Eggplant	390
Kiwifruit	602	Cauliflower	377
Grapes, white	446	Peas, frozen	364
Cantaloupe	252	White potatoes	313
Banana	221	Sweet potatoes	301
Apple	218	Carrots	207
Apricots	164	String beans	201
Peach	158	Tomato	189
Pear	134	Zucchini	176
Watermelon	104	Yellow squash	150

Research tests with mice fed high-ORAC foods found a variety of health benefits in common problems and diseases associated with aging.

1. **Long-Term Memory:** Older and middle-aged ORAC mice exhibited significantly better long-term memory.
2. **Learning Ability:** The ORAC mice retained more of their learning ability as they grew older.
3. **Responsiveness of Brain Cells:** The brain cells of the ORAC mice maintained the ability to respond to chemical stimulus. In mice who received a regular diet, the researchers found that these brain cells had lost forty percent of their ability to respond to such chemical signals by middle age.

4. **Balance and Coordination:** The ORAC mice also had the highest scores in tests designed to measure the brain's ability to maintain balance and coordination.

5. **Capillary Strength:** The small blood vessels (capillaries) of the ORAC mice were much stronger than normal and exhibited less damage and resisted leakage. Decreased capillary strength is associated with strokes and congestive heart failure.

BUY ORGANIC

Whenever possible, you should choose organic fruits and vegetables. The **USDA** recently tested over 27,000 food samples for pesticide residue. One chemical, methyl parathion, accounted for more than ninety percent of the total pesticide residue. The foods found to be the most contaminated were: domestic and imported peaches, grapes, apples, pears, spinach, U.S.-grown green beans and winter squash (both fresh and frozen). Most pesticides tend to be concentrated on or just below the skin on fruits and vegetables, making peeling important. However, foods such as spinach, green beans and squash contain the residue throughout the vegetable.

Even though government authorities assure us pesticides and herbicides are used in safe amounts, the reality is that many of us are already overburdened by toxins from numerous sources. A person whose health is compromised needs to decrease every source of toxicity they can and increase their consumption of "clean" organic fruits and vegetables.

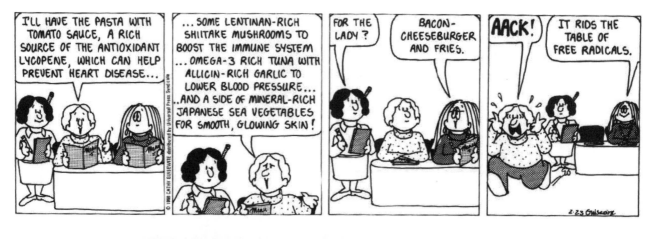

"If we did all the things we are capable of doing,
we would literally astound ourselves."
— Thomas A. Edison

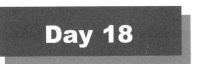

"The future is not some place we are going to, but one we are creating.
The paths are not found, but made,
and the activity of making them
changes both the maker and the destination."

— Pat Conroy

Stimulants are NOT Energy

Stimulants are probably the most common way people self-medicate fatigue. People use a variety of stimulants to "get going" in the morning. Many seniors and Baby Boomers often cannot survive without their morning coffee. Coffee shops flourish with $3 lattes and double-espressos. Gen-Xers and teenagers use their high-octane soda drinks and junk food. Athletes consume drinks with caffeine boosters during their workouts and before events.

Caffeine is one of the most widely used drugs in America because it is so readily available and has widespread social acceptance. "Going for coffee" is considered a symbol of friendship or the basis of many business deals. About eighty percent of U.S. adults drink caffeinated coffee. Some of my clients have reported that they consume two or three **pots** of coffee per day.

Unfortunately, stimulants of all kinds are the least productive ways to achieve energy and are often the most destructive to our energy metabolism. When you consume a stimulant, such as caffeine, the adrenal glands are stimulated to release adrenaline-like substances. These stimulant hormones (glucocorticoids), cause the liver to release sugar and the heart to pump harder. Glucose will be produced from whatever source is available. It may even come from the protein stored in your muscles.

As the blood sugar rises, insulin formation is stimulated in the pancreas in order to bring the blood sugar back down. This creates a biochemical imbalance that often lowers the blood sugar too far, resulting in hypoglycemia, sugar cravings and fatigue. One organ after another is stressed in the effort to maintain body chemistry.

Using the adrenal glands to produce energy from the liver is supposed to be reserved for special circumstances – the "fight or flight" situations. It is a stress response – not something you want to encourage as a daily habit. This type of energy metabolism can rapidly exhaust you by depleting your body of tremendous amounts of nutrients. It is amazing to me how many regular caffeine users are not even taking a multivitamin.

Many people have sought help from a physician for various complaints such as headaches, heart palpitations, high blood pressure, lightheadedness, tremors and anxiety, only to find that their symptoms were relieved when they stopped their caffeine habit. Caffeine is not the innocent little energy booster we think it to be. You should certainly stop using caffeine before you consider taking medications for any of the above complaints. The following chart lists some of the many ways caffeine affects your health.

POTENTIAL HEALTH PROBLEMS FROM DAILY CAFFEINE CONSUMPTION:

- Caffeine stimulates the kidneys, causing dehydration and the loss of many essential vitamins and minerals.

- Caffeine reduces the absorption of iron and calcium from foods and supplements. This increases the risks for osteoporosis and anemia.

- Caffeine increases anxiety, nervousness, panic and chronic fatigue.

- Caffeine raises blood pressure and increases heart rate. Even a five-point increase in diastolic pressure increases the risk of stroke by thirty-four percent and of heart attack by twenty-one percent.

- Caffeine also raises cholesterol and triglycerides.

- Caffeine acts in the body like a pill that stimulates Type A behavior, "exaggerating physical responses to everyday stress," reports James Lane, of **Duke University Medical School** in Durham, North Carolina.

- Caffeine increases the secretion of stomach acid and raises the risk of gastritis, ulcers and heartburn.

- Caffeine increases PMS and menopausal symptoms. It may also increase the frequency of hot flashes.

- Caffeine increases breast pain and contributes to fibrocystic breast disease.

- Caffiene increases Phase 1 liver detoxification (see *Day 25--Love Your Liver*). If the body runs out of nutrients to carry out Phase 2 detoxification, dangerous toxins and drugs can become more toxic than their original form and damage other organs.

CUTTING OUT THE CAFFEINE

Caffeine is a drug that ultimately leads to addiction. Frequent users develop a tolerance for caffeine, suffer withdrawal symptoms, and have cravings for other caffeine-containing products such as chocolate. Caffeine is not something many people can quit "cold turkey." Caffeine withdrawal can cause side effects such as headaches, fatigue and depression. Start decreasing your caffeine intake by one serving per day or as much as a fifty percent reduction each day. If you get a caffeine headache go more slowly.

We have included three charts to inform you of the caffeine content of several foods and beverages. Also note the following ways to overcome caffeine addiction:

- Look for caffeine on labels of foods, beverages and over-the-counter medications. Many headache remedies contain caffeine.
- Decrease your caffeine by making your coffee with half decaf.

- Try coffee substitutes or herbal teas. Green tea has caffeine but can help to wean down your caffeine intake.
- Exercise daily and get plenty of rest.
- Do not skip meals. It will make you think you need caffeine. In reality, your body just needs fuel--eat!
- Avoid chocolate and cocoa, which also have caffeine.

CAFFEINE CONTENT OF COFFEE AND TEA

Beverage	Caffeine Content (in milligrams)
Coffee (7.5-ounce)	
Drip	115+
Brewed	80-135
Instant	65-40
Decaffeinated	3-4
Tea (5-ounce cup)	
1-min. brew	20
3-min. brew	35
Iced (12 ounces)	70
Iced Teas (all 16 oz. Servings)	
Celestial Seasonings Iced Lemon Ginseng Tea	100
Snapple Iced Tea, all varieties	48
Lipton Iced Tea, assorted varieties	18/40
Iced Teas (all 16 oz. Servings) cont...	
Nestea Pure Sweetened Iced Tea	34
Arizona Iced Tea, assorted varieties	15-30
Celestial Seasonings Herbal Iced Tea	0
Flavored Instant Coffees (all 8 oz. Servings)	
General Foods International Coffee, Orange Cappuccino	102
Maxwell House Cappuccino, Mocha	60-65
General Foods International Coffee, Swiss Mocha	55

CAFFEINE CONTENT OF SNACKS AND DESSERTS

Snacks & Desserts	Caffeine Content (in milligrams)
Chocolates and Candies	
Hershey Special Dark Chocolate Bar, 1.5 oz.	31
Hershey Milk Chocolate Bar, 1.5 oz.	10
Coffee Nips hard candy, 2 pieces	6
Hot chocolate, 1 cup	5
Frozen Desserts (1 cup)	
Ben & Jerry's No Fat Coffee Fudge Frozen Yogurt	85
Starbucks Coffee Ice Cream, assorted varieties	40-60
Haagen-Dazs Coffee Ice Cream	58
Healthy Choice Cappuccino Chocolate Chunk Low-Fat Ice Cream	8
Yogurts	
Dannon Coffee Yogurt, 8 oz	45
Yoplait Café Au Lait Yogurt, 6 oz.	5
Dannon Light Cappuccino Yogurt, 8 oz.	<1

According to researchers at **Johns Hopkins Medical Institution** in Baltimore, about seventy percent of soft drinks sold nationwide contain caffeine, and most soda drinkers cannot taste the difference between caffeinated and non-caffeinated drinks. Their study was published in the August, 2000 issue of ***Archives of Family Medicine***.

They concluded that caffeine is added to soft drinks because its addictive nature boosts consumption. Only eight percent of the twenty-five adult cola drinkers tested were able to detect the caffeine in sodas. The **National Soft Drink Asociation** protested that it was a very poorly conducted and designed study.

Apparently Canada does not tolerate any discussion about the merits of caffeine in sodas. They do not allow non-cola soft drinks to contain any caffeine.

CAFFEINE CONTENT OF SOFT DRINKS AND CAFFEINATED WATERS			
Beverage	**Caffeine Content (in milligrams)**	**Beverage**	**Caffeine Content (in milligrams)**
Soft Drinks		*Soft Drinks cont...*	
Jolt	100	Diet Pepsi	36
Jasta	58	Barqs Root Beer	23
Mountain Dew	55	Sprite	0
Surge	51	7 up	0
Tab	47	*Caffeinated Waters*	
Coca-Cola	45	Java Water	125
Diet Coke	47	Krank-2-0	100
Dr. Pepper	41	Aqua Blast	90
Sunkist Orange Soda	40	Water Joe	60-70
Pepsi Cola	37	Aqua Java	50-60

DIET PRODUCTS

Overweight people of all ages are enticed by the slick marketing of "thermogenic" diet products, which feature an herbal stimulant known as Ma huang or ephedra. Radio disc jockeys brag about how many pounds they have lost and how much "energy" they now have after using such products.

Unfortunately, herbal diet stimulants raise your heart rate to unhealthy levels and make your body think it is running an Ultra Marathon all day. Certainly, you will burn more calories but it taxes your heart, thyroid and adrenals. This ultimately leaves your body exhausted and will cause tremendous rebound weight gain when you stop.

Ephedra has been linked to heart attacks, stroke, seizures and death. There have been over eight hundred complaints of side effects, including forty-four deaths. The potential risks far outweigh any temporary benefits.

A chemical cousin to ephedra, known as phenylpropanolamine or PPA, recently was linked to stroke risk. In November, 2000, the **Food and Drug Administration** advised consumers to avoid over-the-counter cold remedies and appetite suppressants with this ingredient. They called on drug companies to stop using it in their products because of a study in the December 21, 2000 issue of *The New England Journal of Medicine*. They estimate products with PPA may be responsible for two hundred to five hundred hemorrhagic strokes (bleeding in the brain) per year, in U.S. adults younger than fifty.

ILLEGAL STIMULANTS

Recreational drug users love the "buzz" of illegal drugs such as cocaine, crack and methamphetamines. They brag about being able to stay awake for several days at a time. These drugs gain power over their victims very fast and are so exhausting the drug user thinks they need more just to function.

The reality of illegal drugs is not fun, but disease, death and destruction. These stimulants are not producing energy. They are comparable to being jolted with electricity! This harassment to your organs causes predictable adverse effects on your health. Many athletes and movie stars who spent time in the fast lane are now having heart attacks in their thirties. Others are having chronic psychiatric problems ranging from depression and panic attacks to schizophrenia.

CASE HISTORY

A few years ago, I had a thirty-five-year-old patient who reported that he had already suffered at least a dozen heart attacks. I asked him why he thought his heart was so weak. He remarked, "Bad genetics, I guess." I then asked him if he had ever used drugs and he replied that he had used methamphetamines for eight years.

I said, "Do you really believe you could use speed for eight years and not have it damage your heart?" He remarked that the heart attacks did not start occurring until he had already stopped his drug use. I explained that damaged organs do not become instantly healthy once you stop abusing them. You have to take steps to nourish the organs back to health to overcome the severe depletion caused by the stimulant. By the way, the illegal drug, methamphetamine, is made from the same ingredient (ephedra) as the thermogenic diet products.

RITALIN FOR DEPLETED KIDS

For years, grade school teachers have been aware of the increased levels of poor behavior and attention spans among many students on the days following "high sugar holidays" such as Halloween and Easter. Now that "candy foods" containing sugar and chocolate have become accepted as breakfast meals, this behavior goes on all year long.

Ritalin is a stimulant drug that has been in use for over forty years to medicate children who are depleted and have subsequent poor brain function. Currently, two million children and adolescents are on Ritalin, an increase of six hundred percent over the past five years according to the **Drug Enforcement Agency**. Americans consume ninety percent of the Ritalin produced worldwide.

Because this drug is a nervous system stimulant, we should be concerned about its long-term health risks. Pharmacologically, it works on the neurotransmitter dopamine, which resembles the stimulant characteristics of cocaine. When taken in accordance with usual prescription instructions, it would be classified as having mild to moderate stimulant properties.

The web site for the **Indiana Prevention Resource Center** at **Indiana University** (**www.drugs.indiana.edu**), has information regarding the latest trend in Ritalin drug abuse involving snorting or injecting crushed pills to produce a strong stimulant effect. Numerous medical journals are reporting permanent and irreversible lung tissue damage related to injection of crushed Ritalin tablets. Snorting has resulted in acid burns to the nasal tissues and deterioration of the nasal cartilage.

Many holistic physicians have helped thousands of children with attention deficits and hyperactivity by helping parents choose a higher quality diet, identifying food allergens and by better nourishing the brain with a high quality multivitamin and omega-3 fats. Cod liver oil comes in several flavors in health food stores. It should not be any more unpleasant giving a child fish oil than it should be to give a dose of Ritalin. Children also need to eat a variety of different vegetables to get their antioxidants, which are so important to brain function. Giving children a "green drink" is another way to build up their alkaline minerals, which are very nourishing to the nervous system.

Dr. William G. Crook has written a book, ***Help for the Hyperactive Child: A Practical Guide Offering Parents of ADHD Children Alternatives to Ritalin***. It is available on his website, **www.candida-yeast.com** or by calling (800) 227-2627. A special feature of this book is a chapter by **Jean Smith, R.N.**, entitled, ***"Feeding Your Child Without Going Crazy."***

TODAY'S ACTIVITY

If you are a regular user of something that produces a stimulant effect, go to the list of caffeine side effects and circle those health problems that you are presently experiencing. Many of these same side effects will apply to all stimulants. Except for the use of prescription medications, plot out your strategy for decreasing your stimulant usage. You should be able to eliminate most products within a period of four weeks:

Present Usage	One Week	Two Weeks	Three Weeks	Four Weeks

Anyone who suffers from frequent fatigue cannot afford to be using stimulants on a daily basis. Some people should not **ever** use stimulants. It is fighting a losing battle to try to build your health while using products that deplete the nutrients that provide you with energy. Stimulating the adrenals to give you "energy" will only exhaust you further and eventually ruin your health. Constantly stimulating the adrenals will increase cortisol production. Cortosol is a nasty hormone when it gets out of control (see ***Day 19--Low Thyroid and Adrenals***).

You cannot produce good quality energy from poor quality food, beverages or drugs. The only way to efficiently produce energy is by converting nutrient-rich food into fuel. If you are tired, eat! If you are still tired, consider the quality of what you are eating.

> "Go confidently in the direction of your dreams.
> Live the life you have imagined."
> — Henry David Thoreau

3 Day Food & Activity Diary

	Date:	Date:	Date:
Morning Meal Time:			
Snack			
Noon Meal Time:			
Snack			
Evening Meal Time:			
Snack			
Symptoms (Physical & Emotional)			
Exercise Type & Duration			

Day 19

"What would you attempt to do if you knew you would not fail?"

— The Rev. Robert Schuller

Low Thyroid & Adrenal Function

Eleven million Americans suffer from low thyroid function (hypothyroidism). One reason it is so prevalent is because of nutritional deficiency. It is next to impossible to get your daily optimal dosage of iodine if you are not taking a multivitamin-mineral. Without adequate iodine, and other nutrient co-factors, your body is unable to make enough thyroid hormone. This eventually causes you to become hypothyroid and require thyroid medication.

The thyroid gland makes hormones that regulate body metabolism and organ function. If your body does not make enough thyroid hormone, you can become tired, depressed and forgetful; which many, including doctors, pass off as "normal" signs of excess stress or aging. Women over fifty years of age are considered most at risk for this disease and have thyroid problems seven times more than men.

In order to produce/synthesize optimal levels of thyroid hormone, you need to have 150 micrograms of iodine in your diet daily. The only significant dietary source of iodine in the typical American diet is shellfish – not regular fish. There is plenty of iodine in kelp and seaweed, but the average American does not consume these foods regularly.

For several decades, Americans have consumed iodized salt. This has greatly decreased the incidence of goiters, but it is usually not enough to provide optimal amounts of thyroid hormone. To exacerbate the problem, there are many Americans who consume no extra salt for fear of making their blood pressure worse. Therefore, the risk of nutritional deficiency causing hypothroidism is still very common.

Selenium is another important mineral for optimal thyroid function. A selenium-containing enzyme (Iodothyronine 5' deiodinase) is responsible for the conversion of thyroid hormone T4 to its active form T3. Both iodine and selenium are ingredients in a good quality multivitamin or prenatal vitamin/mineral supplement.

The thyroid gland can be adversely affected by a cornucopia of other things to which we are commonly exposed. Excessive cortisol function by the adrenals, antidepressant medications, estrogen-containing medications and estrogen-like compounds such as PCB's, dioxins and pesticides can play havoc with an already poorly nourished thyroid gland. Cigarette smoking can produce goiters and increase the severity and metabolic effects of hypothyroidism. Chlorine and sodium fluoride products block iodine receptor sites. Petroleum and coal derivatives are "antithyroid and goitogenic compounds." Even red dye no. 3 can disrupt thyroid hormones.

BEEN TOLD YOUR LAB TESTS WERE "NORMAL"?

So often, people are frustrated because they go to the doctor suspecting they have low thyroid function but are told their blood tests are normal. One reason for this is because the normal values are calculated from an average of the total population who do not have *obvious* hypothyroidism. It is not an average of the most healthy, robust members of our population. Therefore, the undiagnosed cases of low thyroid function alter the normal values. Thus, the blood tests are not very sensitive to the early diagnosis of thyroid problems.

Innovative researcher, **Broda Barnes, M.D.**, wrote a book, ***Hypothyroidism, an Unsuspected Illness.*** In it, he describes how to perform an underarm temperature test, which is a no cost, very sensitive method to confirm early thyroid dysfunction by detecting a decrease in body temperature. If you follow his parameters, you can obtain very accurate results.

Please note: This method recommends using an oral mercury thermometer. However, due to toxicity concerns with broken thermometers, these devices are now either difficult to obtain or not allowed to be sold. **Dr. Barnes'** foundation cautions that inexpensive digital thermometers give unreliable results. The more expensive digital thermometers are more reliable. Using a digital thermometer orally rather than in the armpit may prove more accurate.

THE BASAL BODY TEMPERATURE TEST

1. An oral mercury thermometer should be shaken down to below 96° the night before and left near your bedside where you can reach it easily WITHOUT GETTING OUT OF BED!
2. When you awaken, do not get up or move around a lot. The thermometer should be placed in your mouth or in your armpit against the skin for 10 minutes. Press your arm against your body to hold the thermometer in place. Be sure not to roll over on that side and possibly break the thermometer.
3. For women, if scheduling allows, it is ideal to perform the temperature test on the second or third days after menstruation starts. Your temperature will be naturally higher during ovulation.
4. Do not measure your temperature if you have a cold, sore throat or other infection. Record your temperature to the nearest tenth of a degree (for example, 97.8°).
   Normal armpit temperature is 97.8 to 98.2°F.
   Normal oral temperature is 98.2 to 98.6°F.

Date	Temperature
1. ____	_____
2. ____	_____
3. ____	_____
4. ____	_____
5. ____	_____

Vast research over the past thirty years has linked hypothyroidism to dozens of serious health problems from fatigue and depression to heart disease. Yet, if the hypothyroidism is not addressed, there is no way to improve these conditions. The many symptoms associated with hypothyroidism are listed below:

TODAY'S ACTIVITY

Check if you have some of the common signs of hypothyroidism:

- ❑ Fatigue, especially in the morning
- ❑ Headaches, migraines
- ❑ Weight gain, especially in the hips; fluid retention
- ❑ Slow wound healing
- ❑ Low body temperature and cold intolerance, especially hands and feet
- ❑ Chronic infections, especially during the change in seasons
- ❑ Menopausal problems or menstrual irregularities and heavy flow
- ❑ History of infertility, miscarriages, still births
- ❑ Decreased sex drive
- ❑ Insomnia or narcolepsy
- ❑ Heart problems, hypertension, high cholesterol
- ❑ Dry, coarse skin and hair; brittle nails
- ❑ Hair loss (including outer third of eyebrows)
- ❑ Skin problems, acne
- ❑ Reduced or excessive sweating
- ❑ Poor short-term memory and concentration
- ❑ Depression, crying easily
- ❑ Low motivation, ambition
- ❑ Mood swings, irritability
- ❑ Constipation, acid indigestion, irritable bowel syndrome
- ❑ Deep, hoarse voice, slow speech
- ❑ Pain where the ribs meet the breastbone
- ❑ Muscle and joint stiffness, arthritis

One of the first lab tests to show abnormal low thyroid activity is an elevated TSH. Medical treatment for clinical hypothyroidism is virtually always synthetic thyroid hormone medication, sold under the brand names, Synthroid, Levothyroid, Levoxine, and Levo-T. Symptoms of overdose can include heart irregularities and bone loss. Synthetic thyroid used in combination with various other drugs (anticoagulants, antidiabetic drugs, digitalis, beta blockers, estrogen replacement and oral contraceptive hormones) can cause problems. Once you start on a synthetic hormone, it is usually necessary to use it daily for the rest of your life.

Many alternative physicians recommend a natural thyroid obtained from pigs, known as **Armour Thyroid** (prescription only). This sometimes gets better results because it contains both the T3 and T4 hormones, unlike the synthetic brands, which contain only T4. Many people suffering from hypothyroidism have difficulty converting T4 to the active form of the hormone, T3.

The **Broda Barnes Foundation** is a service organization that will send out educational packets on hypothyroidism. In some cases they will refer you to endocrine doctors who will help you further with remedies such as Armour thyroid. You can visit their web site at **www.BrodaBarnes.org,** or call (203) 261-2101.

Subclinical or mild thyroid imbalances are very common but very few people have the full constellation of symptoms. Some people with subclinical cases of hypothyroid have found success in revitalizing their depressed thyroid gland through the use of specific iodine and non-hormone glandular supplements. You should seek the advice of a nutritionally-oriented doctor rather than trying to figure this out on your own.

If a hair analysis shows extremely low levels of iodine, I often supplement my patients for a few months with a **Metagenics** product called **Energenics**®, in addition to their multivitamin. This product has no thyroid glandular but contains eight nutrients, including iodine, that support thyroid function.

One last note on reasons for hypothyroidism that I have never seen mentioned elsewhere: one of the main functions of thyroid hormone is to keep our bodies and especially our trunks warm. We cannot digest or carry out metabolic functions properly without adequate body heat. This is why people with an underactive thyroid have cold hands and feet. The body is trying to keep as much heat as possible in the trunk.

A bad habit of many Americans is to drink ice-cold beverages with meals and sometimes throughout the day. This causes the thyroid to "work overtime" to constantly try to get the digestive system back to its optimal temperature for all the enzyme reactions to occur. Not only is this a very wasteful use of thyroid hormone, it also increases our requirements for all the nutrients necessary to make it.

ADRENAL FUNCTION

Just like the expression, "Where there's smoke there's fire," a person with abnormal thyroid function often has adrenal gland abnormalities as well. The adrenal glands sit on top of the kidneys and are involved with the mineral "electrolytes" and water excreted or saved during urination. The adrenal glands regulate blood pressure, steroid hormone synthesis and the body's stress mechanism.

The major hormones produced by the adrenals include DHEA, progesterone, cortisol, aldosterone, epinephrine and norepinephrine. DHEA is important to the growth and repair of protein tissues. It is naturally increased by experiencing joy, love, and laughter and by practicing relaxation techniques such as prayer and meditation. It is inhibited by excessive cortisol released during stress.

THE STRESS RESPONSE

Hans Selye coined the term "general adaptation syndrome" to describe a number of biological changes induced by stress. This syndrome has three phases, which are known as alarm, resistance, and exhaustion. All three phases are controlled and regulated by the adrenal glands.

The Alarm Phase is the body's initial response to stress and is often referred to as the "fight or flight" response. The epinephrine hormones (adrenalin) stimulate all parts of our bodies for immediate physical activity. This system goes into action when we experience stresses such as a close call on the freeway, weather disasters, crime or the death of a loved one.

We also voluntarily engage this system when we attend scary or violent movies, go skydiving, ride a roller coaster, play video games, or try bungee jumping. Some people are addicted to this "adrenaline rush" because their bodies have such low energy and vitality. This stressful sensation becomes the only time they feel "alive." When we constantly stimulate our bodies with caffeine, sugar, stimulatory drugs or a stressful lifestyle, we perpetuate this alarm reaction into a state of resistance and eventually exhaustion.

Before exhaustion we experience the Resistance Phase. Resistance continues fighting the stressor long after the alarm stage has worn off. Aldosterone is released to regulate sodium and potassium in order to maintain an elevated blood pressure. Glucose gets depleted during the alarm phase. This causes cortisol hormone, used in the resistance stage, to convert protein to energy.

Many people start their long road to ill health in this stage. The protein broken down for energy often comes from our muscles, leading to muscle wasting, known as sarcopenia. This can be detected by doing a grip strength test or by just feeling the tone of the arms and legs. These muscles feel very soft and remind you of spongecake. The energy metabolism of our muscles can also become severely disrupted during this phase, resulting in the painful muscle condition known as fibromyalgia and its companion condition, chronic fatigue syndrome.

Cortisol helps regulate numerous body functions including glucose metabolism and energy balance. Cortisol is increased by excessive insulin function so it is aggravated by a diet high in refined carbohydrates. Chronic imbalances of this stress hormone can trigger increased fat deposits in the abdomen, leading to the "apple-shaped" obesity associated with a higher risk of type-2 diabetes, heart disease, and stroke.

Cortisol is released during pain and moderates inflammation and immune responses. It often contributes to insomnia and exhaustion in people suffering from painful conditions. When cortisol is decreased, it may cause increased allergy symptoms such as hay fever and asthma. This is especially true of children suffering from severe or persistent attacks and the nocturnal worsening of asthma.

Cortisol also relates to our mental and emotional health. Studies funded in part by the **National Institutes**

of Health on boys, ages seven to twelve, found significantly lower levels of salivary cortisol in those with conduct disorder, characterized by aggressive behavior and disruptive social interactions. Finding an elevated salivary cortisol in the morning has been associated with an increased risk of developing major depression. Adult women had double the risk and teenagers had a seven-fold increased risk in two studies appearing in the **British Journal of Psychiatry**.

The Exhaustion Phase may result in the total collapse of body function or a collapse of specific organs. The major reasons for exhaustion are the loss of potassium ions and depletion of cortisol. Without potassium, cells lose function and eventually die. Without cortisol we cannot adequately maintain our blood sugar and this results in hypoglycemia. This is why people in this state have outrageous cravings for sugar. Unfortunately, sugar will never correct the problem and they continue to spiral downward.

Potassium is found in plentiful amounts in nearly every type of natural food. Seaweeds, nuts, seeds, fruits, vegetables, beans, and meats are great sources. Grains are the poorest sources. Sugar, as I have mentioned in previous chapters, is probably the most depleting "food" on the planet and will never allow our bodies to heal. I hesitate to call sugar a food since it has no nutrients.

In functional medicine, a gradual loss of adrenal function is widely recognized as a contributor to a decline in health. In general, compromised adrenal function will negatively affect one's blood pressure, energy level, sensitivity to allergens and resistance to infection.

When the adrenals are stressed, we use and excrete tremendous amounts of vitamins and minerals. This is why some people who endure a tragedy appear to have their hair turn gray "overnight." The depletion of minerals such as iron, magnesium and copper makes the hair turn gray.

PERSONAL STORY

Adrenal stress not only diminishes your physical vitality, but also your mental and emotional health. Before my mother died, my father was very healthy and active, despite his eighty-one years. Within two months of her death, he lost a great deal of weight and ended up in the hospital with pneumonia. Just a month later, his poor eating habits caused him to become lost and confused while driving. It was in the middle of the winter and darkness brought along a thick fog. He became terrified as he drove for two hours trying to find his way back home. A week later he became lost again and ended up in a ditch. These two stressful events drained his vitality so severely that he became psychotic within a week and had to recover in a psychiatric hospital for six weeks.

Remember this story when you are consuming caffeine, sugar or stimulant drugs, and consider whether your adrenals could withstand the inevitable stresses we all eventually must face. Your adrenals have everything to do with your capacity for resilience. We must keep our adrenals strong to preserve both our physical and mental health. When someone chides me for not wanting to go on roller coasters or try skydiving, I simply reply that I do not pay anyone to stress me out!

Check the following symptoms of low adrenal function to see how you fare:

- ❏ Fatigue, especially in the afternoons
- ❏ Lingering fatigue after exertion
- ❏ Muscle weakness
- ❏ Muscles feel tender, sore or hot
- ❏ Low blood pressure
- ❏ Dizziness when standing up
- ❏ Sensitive to weather changes
- ❏ Mood swings
- ❏ Blood sugar problems
- ❏ Craving salty foods
- ❏ Catch colds easily
- ❏ Large pupils, sensitivity to sunlight

If you checked off many of the adrenal symptoms, you may want to have your cortisol and DHEA tested with the **Adrenocortex Stress Profile** from **Great Smokies Diagnostic Laboratory**. This is a salivary test with four samples taken at home over a twenty-four-hour period to check whether your cortisol is following the normal pattern of rise and fall. For more information on this test visit **www.gsdl.com** or call (800) 522-4762.

Both low blood pressure and big pupils are the result of decreased vascular tone. An adrenal-stressed person will often have the inability to properly close their pupils and will become very sensitive to sunlight. My patients are often surprised how large their pupils appear when I stand next to them in front of a mirror to compare my normal-size pupils to theirs.

The major disease associated with severely decreased adrenal output of the hormone cortisol is called Addison's disease. This requires medical intervention and hydrocortisone medication.

NOURISHING THE ADRENALS

As I mentioned earlier, American Indians would eat the adrenal glands of their freshly killed buffalo. They instinctively knew this would help them recover from the stress of the hunt. Since most Americans no longer kill their own animals, we can build up our adrenals by consuming adrenal extracts from beef in tablet form. Because there are many types of products with different benefits, it is best to seek the guidance of a holistic physician.

Vitamins C, B6, B5 (pantothenic acid), and the minerals zinc and magnesium are the primary nutrients needed for the manufacture of adrenal hormones. They may have to be supplemented for several months in additional amounts over your multivitamin/mineral in order to restore proper adrenal function.

The primary herbs used to improve adrenal function are Licorice root, Ginseng, Ashwaganda, and Astragalus. Licorice root is one of the most highly regarded herbs to treat low adrenal function. It will increase the blood pressure, which is great for those with very low blood pressure but it should be avoided by those with hypertension or who are pregnant. A safe guideline is to avoid exceeding three grams of licorice root per day for more than six weeks.

Metagenics has a product, **Licorice Plus®**, that contains a much stronger dose of licorice root (300 mg. per tablet) than is found in typical store brands. It also contains Ashwaganda, Rehmannia, and Chinese Yam Root. It is best to take this product with an extra source of magnesium and potassium.

Both Siberian and Panax ginsengs are beneficial for adrenal function. The Ayurvedic herb Ashwaganda, also known as "Indian ginseng," is traditionally used for nervous exhaustion and fatigue. Research indicates that Ashwaganda also helps memory and cognition. Few adverse side effects have been reported with prolonged ginseng use and no side effects have been reported with Ashwaganda.

Astragalus is another adaptogenic herb that helps fatigue and adrenal function. I once heard the owner of an herb shop describe how he determined if someone needed Astragalus by the following observation. He said that if the person came in and leaned on the counter and supported himself with his elbows he needed Astragalus.

As I mentioned in a previous chapter, be sure to purchase herbs from a source, such as **Metagenics**, you are sure has been checked for pesticides, herbicides and heavy metals. Many herbs imported from China and India are notorious for these problems. Also, recent investigations on ginseng have reported some products containing fifty percent caffeine on the label instead of one hundred percent ginseng.

"He who cannot rest, cannot work;
he who cannot let go, cannot hold on;
he who cannot find footing, cannot go forward."
— Richard Willard Armour

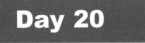

Day 20

"I've learned that no matter how serious
your life requires you to be,
everyone needs a friend to act goofy with."

— Andy Rooney

Stress Management

Stress reduction is crucial to any health program because it can be very toxic and depleting to our health. None of us can totally avoid stress. Therefore we must learn to manage it better. Both physical and psychological stress set off an avalanche of chemical reactions in the body. Depletion occurs when stress hormones mobilize vast amounts of nutrients to create the "fight or flight" response. This is why the outcome of chronic stress is always fatigue and exhaustion.

Poorly managed stress can affect the immune system, heart function, hormone levels, the nervous system, physical coordination, memory and concentration. Some of the health problems associated with stress include mental illnesses, ulcers, bowel disorders, migraines, hypertension, heart disease, cancer, and even the common cold.

Today, nearly one-fifth of all occupational health claims are for job stress. These illnesses cost American businesses some $200 billion per year in medical bills and lost productivity. An October, 2000 study in the **American Journal of Health Promotion**, examined six employers who paid out nearly $20 million a year for eleven modifiable health risks. Of the modifiable health risks such as smoking and obesity, the most expensive lifestyle risk is what employees characterize as "out-of-control" stress. High-level stress accounted for $6.2 million in health costs, compared to $3.2 million for obesity and $2 million for current smokers.

ANGER AND HEART DISEASE

Numerous studies are revealing biological damage to the heart and arteries from anger and hostility. We have been aware for some time that adults who exhibit anger and hostility can experience angina (heart pains) and even heart attacks. Now, research presented at the March, 1999 meeting of the **American Psychosomatic Society**, indicates that cardiovascular disease from hostile emotions can start as early as eight years of age.

Researchers administered personality tests that revealed hostility and measured blood pressure, blood fats and glucose, and body fat. Youngsters with two or more cardiac risk factors, such as high blood pressure and low levels of HDL (beneficial) cholesterol, rated significantly higher in hostility than children with less cardiac risk.

Another study published in September, 1998 in **Psychosomatic Medicine,** showed increased thickening of carotid arteries in middle-aged women who swallowed their anger and were worried about making a positive impression. The lesson to be learned from these two examples is that both inward and outward experiences of anger can be detrimental to the heart. Confronting difficult situations in a more calm, respectful manner can protect your health.

PERSONAL STORY

In my first two years of college, I had to drive an hour each way in heavy, stop-and-go traffic. At first, I would try to "make up time" by darting in and out of lanes, trying to pass as many cars as I could. It did not take long for me to start feeling like a nervous wreck from this stressful commute. I made the decision to start leaving ten minutes earlier every day so I could drive more slowly and not get so tense. Imagine my surprise when I got to school ten minutes early every day. Whether I drove like a maniac or peacefully, the drive took the same length of time!

Even excessive mental thought without emotion is stressful to your heart. A report published in the **Proceedings of the National Academy of Sciences** found that heart patients typically have hyperactivity in the left side of the brain, which is associated with mental calculations and solving math questions. Heart disease patients use less of the right side of the brain.

This would be a strong argument against the "All work, no play" lifestyle. In order to increase activity of the right side of our brains we need to engage in creative activities such as hobbies and music. Meditation, prayer, and breathing exercises also would create more balance between the right and left sides of the brain.

BRAIN DAMAGE FROM STRESS

Chronic stress can cause damage to brain cells in a section known as the hippocampus. But if the high levels of stress discontinue, this area has the unique ability to grow replacement brain cells. MRI studies of Vietnam vets, with post-traumatic stress disorder, showed an average of eight percent smaller hippocampi on the right side of their brains. Survivors of childhood sexual abuse showed twelve percent reduction in the hippocampal size on the left side of their brains.

Patients with depression showed an average of nineteen percent shrinkage of the hippocampus. A group of elderly women, followed over four years, had fourteen percent smaller hippocampi among those whose levels of stress hormones had increased over that time.

PROGRAMMED FOR STRESS

New evidence indicates we are programmed for stress in the womb by the frequency and severity of stress experienced by our mothers. Fetal heart rates jump significantly higher in expectant mothers with the highest levels of stress hormones who reported feeling the most anxiety and the least support. Women with "wanted" babies, who had high self-esteem and ample social support had the calmest fetuses.

In March of 1999, research reported by **Pathik Wadhwa** of the **University of Kentucky College of Medicine in Lexington**, showed that heart rates of fetuses with stressed moms stayed high the longest, suggesting a heightened reaction to stress. Prolonged heart-rate reactions to stress have been linked to a higher-than-normal risk of heart disease and diabetes.

Another study of prenatal stress was done using ultrasound measurements of the fetus' head, abdomen and bone, by **Shalesh Gupta,** of **Cedars-Sinai Medical Center** in Los Angeles. A woman's high stress level retards growth of her fetus, "and the effect is seen as early as the second trimester."

Women with high stress hormone levels were more likely to deliver premature babies. Low birth weight correlates with hypertension in adults and above-average death rates from heart attacks.

RESILIENCE

A positive outlook on life and taking good care of your physical health are key factors to properly managing stress. Everyone's reaction to stress is different. It frequently relates to how we observed our family members handling stress. The important thing to note is that you can make changes in how you react to stress.

Learning to become more resilient to stress is an extremely important lesson. The book, ***The Survivor Personality***, by **Al Siebert, Ph.D**, discusses some of the characteristics needed to better handle stress and change. You can take a quiz entitled, ***"How Resilient Are You?"*** on his web site, **www.thrivenet.com**.

CHARACTERISTICS OF RESILIENCE
Adapted from The Survivor Personality by Al Siebert, Ph.D., used by permission

- Constantly learn from your experience and the experiences of others
- Need and expect to have things work well for yourself and others. Take good care of yourself.
- Adapt quickly and be highly flexible to change.
- Feel comfortable with paradoxical qualities.
- Anticipate problems and avoid difficulties.
- Think up creative solutions to challenges and invent ways to solve problems. Trust intuition and hunches.
- Manage the emotional side of recovery. Grieve, honor and let go of the past.
- Expect tough situations to work out well and keep on going. Help others, and bring stability to times of uncertainty and turmoil.
- Find the gift in accidents and bad experiences.
- Convert misfortune into good fortune.

TODAY'S ACTIVITY

The following is a stress scale that has been created to help you understand how stress from multiple sources can have a compound impact on your health. Check your score to examine your present stress level. Decide which of these can be brought under control in the next year. A total of two hundred or more units in one year increases the likelihood of getting a serious disease.

SOCIAL READJUSTMENT RATING SCALE

Rank	Life Event	Mean Value
1.	Death of spouse	100
2.	Divorce	73
3.	Marital separation	65
4.	Jail term	63
5.	Death of a close family member	63
6.	Personal injury or illness	53
7.	Marriage	50
8.	Fired at work	47
9.	Marital reconciliation	45
10.	Retirement	45
11	Change in the health of family member	44
12.	Pregnancy	40
13.	Sex difficulties	39
14.	Gain of a new family member	39
15.	Business adjustment	39
16.	Change in financial state	38
17.	Death of a close friend	37
18.	Change to a different line of work	36
19.	Increased number of arguments with spouse	35
20.	Large mortgage	31
21.	Foreclosure of mortgage of loan	30
22.	Change in responsibilities at work	29
23.	Son or daughter leaving home	29
24.	Trouble with in-laws	29
25.	Outstanding personal achievement	28
26.	Spouse begins or stops work	26
27.	Begin or end school	26
28.	Change in living conditions	25
29.	Revision of personal habits	24
30.	Trouble with boss	23
31.	Change in work hours or conditions	20
32.	Change in residence	20
33.	Change in schools	20
34.	Change in recreation	19
35.	Change in church activities	19
36.	Change in social activities	18
37.	Small mortgage	17
38.	Change in sleeping habits	16
39.	Change in number of family get-togethers	15
40.	Change in eating habits	15
41.	Vacation	13
42.	Christmas	12
43.	Minor violations of the law	11

Total [   ]

STRESS MANAGEMENT TIPS

Managing stress more efficiently is one of the three major focuses of this entire book. The following is a synopsis of the many ways you can decrease your stress.

- Buy a joke book or rent a funny video and share some chuckles with friends. **Norman Cousins** became famous when he took a unique approach to healing himself from a crippling autoimmune arthritis, known as ankylosing spondylitis. He locked himself in a hotel room with numerous videos of comedy and literally laughed himself well.

- Laughter and joy enhance our body's production of DHEA, which is our anti-stress hormone. It helps counter-act cortisol, a stress hormone that can have numerous destructive influences on our health. A lot of people try to take DHEA hormone in a supplement form but if you do not get rid of your "doom and gloom" attitude, cortisol will still prevail and continue to damage your health.

- Engage in regular exercise. It will increase your energy, relieve tension, and elevate your mood. Find a variety of activities you like and choose something daily to blow off your steam. Even ten or fifteen minutes will greatly enhance how you feel.

- Avoid stimulants that overstress your adrenals. Be aware of the tension produced by exposure to violence in music, television, or video games.

- Take short meditation or breathing breaks throughout the day to calm your mind into an alpha state and tone down the beta brain wave activity.

- Take a class in yoga or tai chi to learn how to become more in touch with how your body holds stress.

- Get regular chiropractic care to help normalize your nervous system's balance from "fight or flight" to "rest and digest!" Do not ignore getting care for "minor injuries." Little pains often accumulate into bigger problems.

- Indulge in a full body therapeutic massage to put your brain and muscles at ease. Make it clear to your therapist that you want very little talking so you will be able to slip into alpha brain wave activity.

- End your workday at a reasonable hour and get a full night's sleep every night. Realize that being overtired is counterproductive to getting your best work accomplished.

- Engage in meaningful relationships. You may not be able choose your relatives, but you can choose your relationships. Avoid people who are abusive or have "toxic" personalities.

- Pets can also provide an extremely valuable daily dose of unconditional love. Studies have confirmed that elderly people with pets live longer and have fewer health problems.

- Find other ways to include valuable relationships in your life. Mentor a child from a troubled home. "Adopt" a senior who never gets visited in a nursing home. Take a special interest in someone who has just experienced the loss of a loved one. Offer to babysit for a single mother.

- Extending your heart to offer love and companionship pays you back very richly. Focusing on love instead of bitterness allows your health and vitality to thrive. Being stuck on past hurts causes your vitality to greatly diminish.

- Learn to express your emotions appropriately. Do not hide from your feelings and stuff your anger. At the same time, avoid spouting off like a volcano, with no consideration for another person's feelings.

- Follow Your Bliss! Find fun in your job and your free time. Numerous studies have found that those who choose a career in alignment with what they are passionate about become much more financially successful.

Last, but not least, eat more slowly. Take time to savor and appreciate your food. Notice how many times you are chewing your food and occasionally make a point to chew thirty times before swallowing. Avoid drinking with your meals so you will be more inclined to chew enough to get adequate saliva with your food. Put your utensils down between each bite to avoid the tendency to continuously shovel more food in.

"Slow Food" is an eleven-year-old anti-fast-food movement, which has forty thousand adherents in thirty-six countries. "Slow Cities," also known as **Città Lente**, is another facet of this movement, now involving thirty-three towns in Italy. They have banded together to preserve Italy's more languid pace, in contrast to the USA's turbocharged economic model. It is becoming more common for people to make conscious choices to get out of the fast lane.

> "To insure good health: Eat lightly, breathe deeply, live moderately, cultivate cheerfulness, and maintain an interest in life."
> — William Londen

Day 21

"You cannot teach a man anything.
You can only help him to find it within himself."
— Galileo

The 5-Minute Meditation Habit

For me, meditation is a topic that fits under the heading of "teach what you want to learn." Meditation is a discipline I have struggled to adapt into my lifestyle for years. I have read books, taken workshops and purchased tapes but still have failed to practice this skill regularly.

I called this chapter the "The 5 Minute Meditation Habit" because I felt that the most I could ask of anyone who is struggling to make changes in their health and lifestyle is five minutes out of each day. If I were tell someone the only way for them to consider meditating is to devote at least twenty minutes, most people would not even attempt it. That just seems like too much time and effort for many of us.

When I first started writing this book, I was meditating at least once and often twice per day. Many of my meditations lasted twenty minutes or more. It was easy. I had the house to myself and my time was my own. But then my son returned home from visiting his dad for five weeks and my whole routine was rearranged.

At least that is my excuse. How could I not find five minutes in every day? After all, I am not with my son twenty-four hours per day. The truth is, most of us have an important health habit that we find excuses to avoid doing regularly. For many, this stumbling block is physical exercise. Whether it is physical or mental exercise, many of us have a belief that we cannot afford the time.

Perhaps if I meditated regularly, the reason for my avoidance would become painfully obvious. In fact, I am sure it would. I have often gone into a meditation with a question I want my brain to figure out. The answer often pops up in less than five minutes. Imagine that! It does not take very long.

People have been using meditation for centuries to unlock the mysteries of life. Many of our great inventions have come about from the practice of meditation. It has helped unlock the creativity that enables people to solve mathematical equations and produce great works of art. By all accounts, it makes us more productive. It certainly does not rob time from our day. If anything, it stops us from "spinning our wheels."

Dr. Herbert Benson, of **Harvard**, wrote about the scientific evidence that supports the many health benefits of meditation in his groundbreaking book, ***The Relaxation Response***. Research is making it crystal clear that every health problem involves stress of some kind. Regularly employing multiple methods of stress reduction, such as meditation, is crucial to gaining control over your health.

BIOFEEDBACK

If you have difficulty calming your mind, you may want to try biofeedback. Start with the guidance of a trained practitioner because there are several techniques available. Various types of equipment measure heart rate, brain-wave patterns, muscle activity, skin temperature or perspiration levels. Your practitioner will help you find the method that works best for you.

A biofeedback device gives "feedback" as sounds or images on a machine or a computer screen. The feedback trains your body and mind to employ stress-reducing techniques to create a more desirable state of relaxation. Eventually you will be able to use these techniques to achieve the same state without the equipment. The average course of treatment is five to twenty sessions. Some disorders may take longer. You may also be able to obtain devices to practice daily at home.

For more information about biofeedback or to locate a practitioner in your area, call the **Association for Applied Psychophysiology and Biofeedback** at (800) 477-8892, or visit **www.aapb.org**.

MEDITATION TAPES AND CLASSES

Using a tape to guide you through meditation is a great way to escape and unwind. Look for tapes of varying length so you can pick and choose, depending on how much time you can devote each day. Finding good tapes for meditation is as easy as going to your local bookstore. You can also try specialty and online bookstores and churches.

An excellent recording of meditations combined with beautiful music and guided imagery, was released in 1997 by **Dr. Andrew Weil**. It is called **"Eight Meditations for Optimum Health."** The meditations range in length from six to ten minutes and are excellent to listen to in sequence. The topics of his meditations include self-healing, self-love, conscious eating, beauty, loving kindness and connectedness. It is available in major bookstores.

Another outstanding source for a wide variety of tapes on meditation and mind-body healing is **Learning Strategies Corporation** in Minnesota, (800) 735-8273, **www.learningstrategies.com.** They offer a recording on deep relaxation and others that focus on improving health, memory, anxiety, negative beliefs, and weight problems. They also have a recording to help quit smoking.

After you have listened to a few professional recordings, you may want to compose your own in order to insert affirmations and music that are most meaningful to you. I would also encourage you to try group meditations or invite some friends to get together every week as "prayer partners." I have been involved in several prayer groups over the years and have received tremendous benefit from these experiences.

TODAY'S ACTIVITY

MEDITATION

First, consider some activity you are presently doing that interferes with the time you will need to dedicate to the daily practice of meditation. That one is easy for me. When I sit down to write at my computer, I rationalize that playing a few computer games first will sharpen my brain and help me organize my thoughts. Write your primary procrastination method or avoidance device here: _____

Start meditating either in the morning or before bed. Find a comfortable chair or a special location in a room that you will designate as your meditation area. Be sure to wear loose, comfortable clothing.

Begin with a short prayer. Use your prayer as a means of surrendering to your highest good. Next do some breathing techniques. When you no longer need to count breaths, start silently pondering an important question. Phrase it by stating the problem and leave it open like a fill-in-the-blank sentence. Try to state the problem in positive terms related more to the outcome you desire, such as:

"The most important thing that will improve my energy today is _____."
NOT: "The main reason I am tired is _____."

If after several days, your question is not producing an answer, state it another way. Consider something like, "I am vibrantly healthy and energetic, therefore, _____
_____."

You may want to write down some of the answers that come to you. This may allow you to uncover an emotional conflict that you would be compelled to face if you had good health.

> "There are no mistakes, no coincidences,
> all events are blessings given to us to learn from"
> — Elisabeth Kübler-Ross

3 DAY FOOD & ACTIVITY DIARY

	Date:	Date:	Date:
Morning Meal Time:			
Snack			
Noon Meal Time:			
Snack			
Evening Meal Time:			
Snack			
Symptoms (Physical & Emotional)			
Exercise Type & Duration			

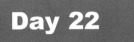

The Energetics of Food

One of the most valuable tools I have learned from studying Oriental Medicine and the Macrobiotic diet is an understanding of the type of energy we receive from food. This knowledge will help you gain power over both your physical energy and your mental/emotional health.

The person who most inspired me to learn more about the Macrobiotic diet was **David Briscoe,** who is now doing macrobiotic health counseling in California. In the 1980's, I had the good fortune of opening my first chiropractic office in Kansas City, upstairs from a Macrobiotic restaurant operated by David and his wife, Cynthia.

David has an interesting history. He cured himself of schizophrenia using only the macrobiotic diet and no nutritional supplementation. David suffered from mental illness most of his childhood, and was on the drug Thorazine for six years. Within a year of eating higher quality foods he was able to get off his medication forever. He has lived a normal life without psychiatric drugs for nearly thrity years. He and his wife have six children and both teach the Macrobiotic eating principles. They offer Macrobiotic home-study programs through their web site **www.macroamerica.com**, or by calling (877) 622-2637.

I think of David whenever I hear of the explosion of ADD, ADHD and mental illnesses such as depression and bipolar disorders among Americans. The reason these conditions are becoming rampant is because nutrient depletion is much more common due to the many factors already discussed in this book.

Many doctors consider these disorders to be incurable and drug-dependent because they are not taught nutritional interventions. The good news is that most of the people suffering from these conditions can achieve a much higher level of functioning if they apply nutrition and Macrobiotic eating principles to their therapeutic regimes. Making diet changes may *eventually* help to decrease or eliminate the need for drugs.

Please Note: Do not ever stop or decrease your medications without the advice of your physician. Improving mental and physical health with diet and nutrition takes time.

David is living proof that nourishing the brain with high quality, nutrient-rich foods can heal the "biochemical imbalances" which are essentially malnutrition of the brain. Many more people like him can be converted from a life of mentally disability to being a productive member of society.

Please do not misconstrue that I am saying everyone can eventually get off psychiatric drugs if they follow this advice. Some people have suffered too much oxidative damage to their brains and will need drug therapy forever. This is especially true with some elderly patients, people who have used multiple medications, those who have abused alcohol and illegal drugs, and victims of chemical or other toxic exposures. David was still young when he made his changes and a complete recovery was possible for him.

My most important message is that people with mental illnesses will never achieve their maximum level of balance and stability with drugs alone. Drugs will never cure a depleted brain because they do not replace vital nutrients needed for its proper function. You always have to consider the nutritional status of the patient.

Mental health treatment needs to shift its focus from treating patients as victims who have no power over their condition. Teaching people to take responsibility for restoring their minds and bodies with better health habits is mandatory to enable them to overcome depletion and improve energetic balance. Those in psychiatric hospitals who are too ill to care for themselves should be fed nutritious meals devoid of sugar, caffeine and junk food. Nutritional supplementation with multivitamins, antioxidants and essential fats ("The Big 3") should become the minimum standard of care for everyone whose condition is severe enough to require medication.

Psychologists need nutritional training to determine whether nutritional depletion is impacting those they are counseling. Many clients with mild stress disorders will recover faster and more completely when they are better nourished. No amount of counseling will overcome a poorly functioning, nutrient-deficient brain.

EXPANSION AND CONTRACTION

There is no way to explain the energetics of food without using the terms expansion and contraction, often described with the terms yin and yang. Over the years of teaching this concept I have often been surprised when some people have a religious conflict discussing the meaning of these terms. Being a Christian, I can assure you that in nearly twenty years of studying Oriental Medicine, I have never been exposed to Eastern religions and therefore have nothing to teach on the subject. Please keep an open mind about these concepts. I have seen this information offer tremendous benefits to hundreds of people.

The concept of expansion and contraction is fundamental to understanding Oriental medicine. These ideas developed from observing nature and its grouping into pairs of mutually dependent opposites. For instance, there is neither night without day, nor cold without hot.

Contraction represents male energy and expansion is female energy. However, each of us has characteristics of both male and female. A healthy man exhibits female traits such as compassion and creativity. A healthy female exhibits male energy qualities such as strength and analytical thinking. When a man or woman needs to build characteristics of male or female energy, they can do so by choosing foods that nourish those qualities

It is interesting how we have always characterized certain foods as male or female. We even have an expression, "Real men don't eat quiche." Eating meats and game are thought to be manly, while eating salads and fruits are considered more popular among women.

It was recently reported that vegetarians give birth to more girls. Since meats produce male energetic qualities this is no surprise. Vegetarians can build a diet with more male energy if they understand the energetics of their food. People often try to guess the baby's gender by looking at the shape of the woman's tummy. The more contractive males look like a big basketball, all out front. You are often unable to discern if a woman carrying a boy is pregnant if observed from behind. More expansive female babies cause the expectant mother to look very broad.

PERSONAL STORY

A few months after I gave birth to my son, I opened my first also chiropractic office. Giving birth is definitely a strong "female energy" event. Any new mother will tell you that for the first several months after giving birth it is very hard to do analytical tasks. We call it "Mommy brain." Here I was trying to start a new business, which is definitely a "male energy" project. It is almost comical to recognize now why I was so ravenous for meats at the time. I was subconsciously trying to build up my male energy.

The **Standard American Diet** is an excellent example of an extreme expansive diet. Americans are both taller and heavier than most other cultures and both of these characteristics can lead to premature death. Asian people are both shorter and less prone to obesity when they eat the more contractive and balanced foods in their traditional diets.

Eliminating expansive refined carbohydrates is a primary reason for the success of the very popular high protein diets. Protein is very contractive and builds muscle. Refined carbohydrates get converted into fat, which is definitely expansive. Eating too much from the strong contractive category without balancing it with plenty of balanced foods actually causes you to crave foods from the strong expansive category. The chart below and on the following page will help you better understand the differences between the expansive and contractive properties of foods and cooking methods.

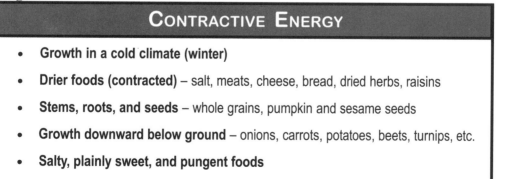

CONTRACTIVE ENERGY

- **Growth in a cold climate (winter)**
- **Drier foods (contracted)** – salt, meats, cheese, bread, dried herbs, raisins
- **Stems, roots, and seeds** – whole grains, pumpkin and sesame seeds
- **Growth downward below ground** – onions, carrots, potatoes, beets, turnips, etc.
- **Salty, plainly sweet, and pungent foods**
- **Frying, baking, or grilling**

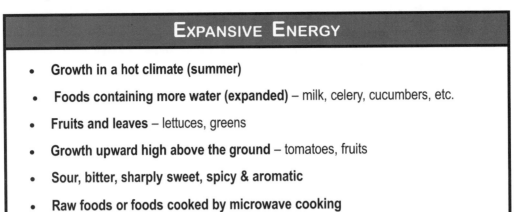

EXPANSIVE ENERGY

- **Growth in a hot climate (summer)**
- **Foods containing more water (expanded)** – milk, celery, cucumbers, etc.
- **Fruits and leaves** – lettuces, greens
- **Growth upward high above the ground** – tomatoes, fruits
- **Sour, bitter, sharply sweet, spicy & aromatic**
- **Raw foods or foods cooked by microwave cooking**

The Macrobiotic diet teaches that we need to vary our diet with the seasons, and primarily eat foods that are grown locally and in season. In the wintertime we naturally gravitate toward contractive energy foods such as stews, and soups made with proteins and root vegetables like carrots, onions and potatoes. Northern climate populations eat a great deal more fish and meat than places closer to the equator. Casseroles, chili and meatloaf are most popular during the winter months, but generally feel too heavy for the summertime.

When the weather is hot, we tend to consume more raw foods like salads and fresh fruits, and crave sweeter foods like juices and ice cream. We are more likely to desire a protein shake for breakfast, rather than bread and baked goods. We eat smaller portions of meat and often serve grilled meat on top of salads. Cooked vegetables such as mashed potatoes and thick soups lose their appeal.

Fruits like bananas, citrus, mangos and pineapples should be consumed primarily by people who live in the hot climates where they are grown. Apples, peaches, etc. are more appropriate for those living in cooler climates. A fruit's expansive energy can be made more contractive by cooking it, such as baked apples or fried bananas.

ENERGETIC QUALITIES OF FOODS

Strong Contractive Foods: Refined salt, eggs, meat, cheese, poultry, fish, seafood, blue-green algae

Balanced Foods: Whole grains, seeds, beans and bean products, nuts, sea vegetables, spring or well water, root, round and leafy vegetables, nonaromatic, nonstimulant teas, natural sea salt

Strong Expansive Foods, etc.: (In ascending order of mild to excessive) Fruit, white rice, white flour, tropical fruits & vegetables, milk cream, yogurt, oils, spices & aromatic herbs, stimulants - coffee, black tea, chocolate; honey, sugar & refined sweeteners; alcohol, food chemicals, preservatives & dyes, pesticides; medications (tranquilizers, antidepressants, etc.), illegal drugs (marijuana, cocaine, methamphetamines, PCP, etc.)

The principles of expansion and contraction relate to everything from our internal body chemistry to our external behavior. If a person suffers from internal contraction such as high blood pressure, asthma, or constipation they should eat less foods in the strong contractive foods category. The magnesium and other minerals found in the chlorophyll-rich leafy vegetables provide the expansion that helps relieve these conditions.

People in Northern climates (contracted behavior) tend to be quieter and more reserved than those in tropical environments who are more exuberant and outgoing (expansive behavior). If you would like to overcome shyness, tone down the contractive foods in your diet and eat more balanced and expansive like salads and greens. Many people have used alcohol (a strong expansive) to temporarily overcome their shyness.

Excessive alcohol is well-known for inhibiting an individual's self-control. People who regularly consume excessive alcohol or drugs can be so expansive in their behavior that they disrespect the boundaries of others and can take on criminal or violent tendencies.

Overly expansive people also have more difficulty organizing their lives and realizing their goals. This is why alcohol and illegal drug users tend to drop out of school, quit jobs, hop from one thing to the next and can become non-productive and homeless. Alcoholics and drug addicts not only have difficulty caring for themselves, but they also often neglect or abuse their children. I cringe when I hear about all the coffee and donuts being served at **Alcoholics and Narcotics Anonymous** meetings.

EFFECTS ON BEHAVIOR OF EXTREME EXPANSIVE OR EXTREME CONTRACTIVE FOOD:

Overexpansion	Overcontraction
Too open, "spaced out"	Too tense, "uptight"
Vague and impractical	"Control freaks"
Too open & permissive	Too strict
Too expressive	Too withdrawing
Overly impressionable	Overly discriminating
Give away their power	Want to overpower others
Poor boundaries	Overstep others boundaries
Seem lazy or confused	Overly rigid and inflexible
Disorganized	Very organized

Addiction behaviors nearly always involve something that produces excessive expansion and will never be cured while consuming an alternate form of expansion such as sugar and caffeine. This is why alcoholics and drug addicts feel so powerless over their conditions. Strongly depleting foods like sugar and caffeine rob you of your personal power and inner strength. You do not help people who feel powerless by baking them cookies.

Recreational drugs are often described as "mind expanding." I have seen many patients who were former drug users who suffer from permanent mind expansion. They often struggle with depression, anxiety, panic attacks and schizophrenia and require prescription medications to function. Now there is proof of this permanent damage visible on brain scans of drug users. The **National Institute on Drug Abuse's** web site, **www.drugabuse.gov,** shows abnormal brain scans of drug users supplied by **Johns Hopkins University.**

To overcome an expansive condition, you will gain tremendous power over your physical and mental/ emotional health by eating more contractive and balanced foods. Most people think of Macrobiotics as a vegan diet, but if you are recovering from years of excessive expansion it can be considered Macrobiotic to eat animal and fish protein.

Blue green algae, of the ***Aphanizomeon flos-aquae*** variety, is a fantastic food for nourishing the brain when there is excessive expansion. It has twenty amino acids in nearly the exact proportions found in our bodies. It also has the essential fatty acids that are so important to our brain function. In the five years I have consumed the algae, I have noticed much more mental clarity and the ability to focus on my goals. I have used this product (specifically **Omega Sun®**) with numerous people who have learning and memory problems. The **Alpha Sun®** product is used to improve physical energy.

Cell Tech Inc., the major distributor of blue green algae from Klamath Falls, Oregon, has seen tremendous improvement in the mental capacities of different groups of impoverished children throughout the world who have received their donations of **Super Blue Green® Algae**. They have worked the longest with one group from Nicaragua. At the beginning, this group was so malnourished they did not have the energy to play. Their school test scores were the worst in their entire country. In recent years this group was tested again and found to have the best test scores in their nation.

TODAY'S ACTIVITY

1. Check the chart on "The Energetic Qualities of Foods," and circle those items you use at least three times per week. Identify the areas where the majority of your diet is.
2. Note the "Behavior Characteristics" chart, and circle those items that apply to you.
3. Identify ways to change your diet to achieve more balance.

Eating foods from the strong expansive or contractive food categories is not necessarily bad. Just understand that you cannot consume excessive amounts in either category without throwing your physical and mental health out of balance. Consuming the majority of your foods in the balanced category can pay tremendous dividends for your energy and emotional health.

One of my favorite descriptions of how eating with the macrobiotic principles can affect your health and behavior comes from **Michio Kushi** in ***The Cancer Prevention Diet***: "With proper eating on the ***Cancer Prevention Diet***, it normally takes the blood plasma ten days to change in quality. Within this period the patient should experience relief in digestive and respiratory functions as well as disappearance of bodily pain. After about two weeks on the diet, circulatory and excretory changes are felt, the emotions begin to change, and the patient will generally feel less depressed and less angry. Nervous functions improve after about one month and thinking tends to become clearer and more focused. After three to four months, the body's red blood cells have completely changed in quality, and the skin, bones, organs, and tissues begin to heal. At this time the person's relations with family and friends often become gentler, more respectful, and loving. Nervous cells take three seasons or approximately nine months to alter, and after this time the person's view of life may become broader, more flexible and more understanding."

I have seen this progression of healing in countless patients over the years. Understanding the energetics of food certainly is an example of the idea that "you are what you eat." Changing your diet to improve the effect on your physical and mental energy can noticeably improve your quality of life. It is most rewarding when parents get to discover their calm and peaceful child who was previously overshadowed by hyperactivity and tantrums. They are thrilled when teachers and family members remark about the improvement in their child's behavior.

My personal sense of power has increased greatly by following macrobiotic principles. It is much easier for me to confront adversity, rather than cave in from it. I am much more direct with others, and not afraid to handle disagreements.

MICROWAVE ENERGY

I would like to end with a warning about microwave cooking. This is the least desirable form of cooking and should be avoided whenever possible. Microwave energy drastically changes the energetic quality of foods by exploding the water molecules in your food to create heat. This extreme expansive energy can create the excessive yin behavior characteristics listed previously.

Unfortunately, many fatigued and depressed people feel too tired to cook, and eat nothing but microwave frozen meals. Hopefully, this chapter will help you understand how that type of food contributes to these problems. You will never overcome fatigue and emotional disorders until fresh, high vitality natural foods are added to the diet. It does not take long to cook greens or stir-fry meals. They are well worth the effort.

The other type of microwave energy we need to be concerned about is the microwave signals emitted from cordless and cellular telephones. England is leading the way in cautioning against allowing children to use these devices. I agree with them that we need to stress prevention of possible health consequences, rather than waiting for frightening statistics to be collected. I personally do not use a cordless phone and only rarely use a cell phone. If you insist on using such devices, by all means get a headset that plugs into your phone so you do not put the strong microwave signal next to your head.

> "You don't have to cook fancy or complicated masterpieces–
> just good food from fresh ingredients."
> — Julia Child

Day 23

"As for butter versus margarine,
I trust cows more than chemists."
--Joan Gussoc, Assistant Professor of Nutrition and Education,
Teacher's College, Columbia University

Good Fats, "Bad" Fats & HORRIBLE Fats

Once upon a time, there were no good or "bad" fats. The fats found in natural foods are absolutely essential to every cell, and therefore, are called "*essential* fatty acids." Our bodies are designed to ingest fats, with different functions, to provide balance in our body's metabolism. The trouble with fats began when man started inventing new ways to alter the fats in foods for a longer "shelf-life."

Partially hydrogenated oils ("trans" fats) do not exist in natural foods. They are processed versions of naturally occurring fats and oils. "Cis" and "trans" refer to molecular shapes of fats that are mirror images of each other. Hydrogenation of plant oils for solidification is produced by adding a nickel catalyst, heating them, passing hydrogen through them, re-bleaching them, and then removing the nickel catalyst by filtration.

The difference between cis and trans shapes is very significant. When eaten, fats and oils are incorporated into *every one* of your cell membranes. Trans fats alter the configuration of these delicate structures. When trans fats interact with normal fat metabolism, they disturb this function in a most destructive manner. *Hence, these substances meet the medical definition of a poison.* **Dorland's Medical Dictionary** defines "poison" as, "any substance which, when relatively small amounts are ingested...has chemical action that may cause damage to structure or disturbance of function, producing symptomatology, illness or death."

Trans fats interfere with important, normal body functions. They inhibit enzymes, which are necessary for proper metabolism of fats, and they continue doing it for a long time. When you eat normal cis fats, your body metabolizes half of them in eighteen days. When you eat trans fats, your body requires fifty-one days to metabolize half of them. This means half of the trans fats you eat today will still be inhibiting essential enzyme systems in your body fifty-one days from now.

Read labels as if your life depended on it because it does! Partially hydrogenated (trans) oils are found in a majority of grocery store products to give the food a longer shelf life and to solidify liquid fats. Because this is so important to your well-being, health food stores commonly carry similar, alternative products that prominently state "No hydrogenated fats" on their labels. Health food stores also tend to carry a higher quality of liquid vegetable oils. You should look for oils that claim to be "cold-pressed." Using heats or solvents to extract oils from plants degrades the oil. Buy small quantities of oil and keep them refrigerated.

<table><tr><td>

TODAY'S ACTIVITY

SOURCES OF HYDROGENATED FATS

Check labels and note which of the following foods in your diet contain trans or partially hydrogenated fats. Read labels and look in your cupboards and refrigerator for other foods not mentioned here:

- ❑ Margarine
- ❑ Vegetable shortenings
- ❑ Chocolate, carob chips, and candy
- ❑ Bread and breadcrumbs
- ❑ Crackers
- ❑ Cookies, snack cakes, etc.
- ❑ Snack foods – chips, pretzels, etc.
- ❑ Other

- ❑ Nuts and sunflower seeds
- ❑ Commercial peanut butter
- ❑ Coffee creamers
- ❑ Fancy coffees & hot chocolate
- ❑ Microwave popcorn
- ❑ Frozen dinners
- ❑ Canned soups

</td></tr></table>

It is preferable to buy whipped butter in tubs because stick butter can have hydrogenated fats. Hydrogenation makes fats harder so butter sticks retain their shape better. It is also what gives chocolate chips and candy their shape. Carob chips (an alternative to chocolate) may also be made with hydrogenated fats.

Check labels on commercial brands of nuts for hydrogenated fats . The best way to purchase nuts is in their shell. Once a nut has been removed from its shell the fats start to become rancid. When buying shelled nuts, select those in their whole form. Every cut surface of a nut can suffer rancidity to the oils. I prefer to buy whole nuts and seeds at a health food store that bags and refrigerates them to retain freshness. Many health food stores also have a peanut-grinding machine to make freshly ground peanut butter, on demand. Buy only what you can finish in a month and keep it refrigerated.

When stir frying, use "extra virgin" olive oil. This is the first press of the olives, which is extracted without chemical solvents. Virgin and pure olive oils are much lower in quality. Olive oil is an omega-9 oil and has the highest "flash point" of vegetable oils. This means it can be heated at a higher temperature before it degrades. Buy olive oil in small quantities and keep in a closed cupboard. It is very sensitive to air and light, which is why gallons of olive oil are sold in metal cans. Most other oils should be stored in the refrigerator.

THE IMPORTANCE OF OILS

Many essential functions in our bodies depend on a group of hormones called prostaglandins (PG's), which are produced from fats in our diets. In a general sense, there are good PG's and "bad" PG's. Most of the ill effects of chronic disease are promoted by or aggravated by an overabundance of "bad" PGs called the PG 2 family. These include: heart attacks and strokes, cardiovascular disease, arthritis, cancer, benign cysts and tumors, neurological diseases, inflammatory conditions and autoimmune diseases. The PG 2 family is derived directly from naturally occurring fat that is found in red meat, shellfish and dairy products.

Nature has devised two other prostaglandins to counterbalance PG 2. They are omega-6 oils, which produce PG 1, and omega-3 oils, which produce PG 3. Omega-6 oils are found in corn, safflower, sunflower and peanut oils. Omega-3 oils are EPA and DHA which come from fish, algae, walnuts and flax seed oil.

Trans fats block good PG 1 production, and by default, the bad PG 2 substances are produced unopposed. Some of the symptoms that are created by good PG's being blocked include headaches, depression, joint pains, back pain, arthritis, asthma, skin problems (rashes, acne and cancers), hot flashes, PMS, menstrual cramps and irregularity, and problems with nerve transmission occurring with diseases such as Multiple Sclerosis.

PERSONAL STORY

My child is one of few kids in America who has no memory of his mother baking chocolate chip cookies for him. What a deprived child! He also has no memory of being rewarded for good behavior with candy. He has never had his concept of love distorted by sugar or other unhealthy foods.

My son does, however, have many memories of me cooking nutritious meals for him. He will also remember me making birthday desserts with healthy ingredients. His association of food and love is of me making every effort to teach him how to choose foods that will help him be strong and healthy.

I am not saying he never eats chocolate or other sugar foods. He consumes them on occasion with the full knowledge that they cause depletion and have the potential to cause health problems. Whenever he develops a cold or other infection he knows to avoid such foods so his body can become stronger and heal.

In my practice, I have seen many women over the years who have had menstrual irregularities or other menstrual difficulties their entire lives. My first question is always, "Did you grow up using margarine?" The answer has been yes at least ninety-five percent of the time. The other five percent had some other major source of hydrogenated fats they consumed regularly, such as chocolate.

Our entire hormonal function depends on normal fat metabolism. If these abnormal, trans fats take over and impact every cell, tissue, and organ, we are guaranteed to develop abnormal function and diseases. We cannot underestimate the devastating impact trans fats have had on our health.

Cancer used to affect one in forty people at the turn of the century. Now it affects one in three. Neurological diseases and hormonal dysfunctions are rampant. Painful conditions such as arthritis and fibromyalgia are escalating at a rapid rate. Fibromyalgia was not even a known disease twenty years ago, when I was studying medicine. Arthritis is affecting many people at much younger ages. Joint replacement surgeries are now commonly done on people in their fifties instead of their eighties.

Heart disease is still the number one cause of death. Consider my frustration over the years trying to convince my patients with heart disease to avoid margarine when their cardiologist was telling them the opposite. Patients then became frustrated and confused when the medical profession finally began to recant that advice after at least forty years of promoting the use of margarine.

It sometimes takes years for important scientific data to become common knowledge because the information seems to be downplayed if it cuts into a powerful food industry's bottom line. Just look at how **Oprah Winfrey** was crucified by the beef industry for doing a show on **Mad Cow Disease**. Some of the American food industries pitched major fits when they were not favorably portrayed on the FDA food pyramid. Before the medical profession started cautioning people about trans fats, every news story about trans fats hazards included the disclaimer, ***"More research is needed."***

ARE YOU "FAT PHOBIC?"

The next issue we need to discuss is "Fat Phobia." This is the mistaken belief that eating fat makes you fat and avoiding fat makes you thin. After a solid decade of full-fledged fat phobia, we can definitively say this thinking is a huge myth. The fat-phobic 1990's produced the biggest increase in obesity of any decade. It is obviously not just fat making us fat. I have seen some patients who were so fat-deficient that they were developing hormonal problems, their hair was falling out or they were developing a neurological disease.

One of the big problems if you are not eating fat or properly digesting and absorbing fat is that you will not be able to properly absorb the fat-soluble vitamins (A, D, E, and K). This is also a concern when you are taking fat-blocking drugs such as cholesterol medications. If you do not absorb vitamin D, you will not be able to properly utilize calcium and your bones will suffer. Lack of vitamin A affects the health of your eyes, skin, lungs and intestines. Deficient E and K affect cardiovascular health.

Fat Phobia is closely related to another myth, "The only way to lose weight is to cut calories and increase exercise." Increasing exercise is certainly important. However, the way you look and feel has everything to do with the quality of what you put into your mouth; not a number relating to calories or fat grams. You cannot eat garbage and feel like anything but garbage. You will start to feel more energy and vitality when you eat high quality foods and engage in a healthy lifestyle. This includes clean water, pure air, adequate rest and recreation. I have witnessed numerous people who exercise fanatically but are unable to lose weight because they are eating foods that create insulin resistance (see ***Day 5--The Sugar Blues***).

The never-ending parade of diets and diet-product fads is a strong indicator that the obese population is being taken for a big ride. I will share with you several important strategies for successful weight management I have employed in my own life for twenty-five years. In that time I have never struggled with weight and have helped numerous patients achieve healthy weight loss. If you make a point to consume good, quality food, you can eat heartily.

The following list of dietary tips will put a healthy perspective on the subject of weight control. Remember, the goal of losing weight is to become healthier, not damage your health, which is becoming far too common.

HEALTHY TIPS FOR WEIGHT MANAGEMENT

- **Skip low fiber foods** – Avoid refined breads, sweets and pasta. Eat plenty of the lower carbohydrate fruits and vegetables – especially dark green leafy vegetables. Remember: "Green inside is clean inside."
- **You will never lose weight if you are constipated** – A toxic bowel creates a sluggish liver – the very place where we metabolize our fats! Laxatives and "diet teas" only weaken the bowel. High protein, *low* vegetable diets are a good recipe for colon cancer. Eat *lots* of vegetables and moderate amounts of fruit and beans to bring moisture to the bowel. Be sure to ingest adequate bacteria (*acidophilus* and *bifidus*) so your bowel will be able to ferment these fibers. Protein and vegetable diets with only *complex* carbohydrates are fine.
- **Eat good fats!** – Healthy dietary fats are essential for proper fat metabolism. A low-fat diet usually has too many pastas, breads and sweets, all of which cause insulin dysregulation and prevent you from burning fat for energy.
- **Avoid consumption of partially hydrogenated or trans fats** —Keep in mind, these are much harder to eliminate and metabolize than natural fats.
- **Steer clear of "Herbal Speed" - Ma huang or ephedrine diet products** – Stimulation is not the same as energy. These products severely tax the heart and adrenals. They cause you to lose nutrients that can contribute to heart attacks, stroke, hypertension, depression, rebound weight gain, etc.
- **Artificial sweeteners** – These have never been proven to help anyone lose weight. Aspartame contains methanol, which is a dangerous neurotoxin and liver toxin. If you disrupt liver function, it will be more difficult for your body to properly metabolize fats. Remember: "If God didn't make it, don't eat it!"
- **Avoid excessive consumption of expansive foods and cooking methods (microwave)** – (See *Day 22--The Energetics of Food*). This chapter discusses how refined sugars, carbohydrates, dairy, alcohol, stimulants and artificial ingredients affect your health and create expansion (weight gain). Dairy foods are designed to make big, strong calves and they tend to make humans hefty.
- **See a holistic physician to determine if you have food allergies caused by a "leaky gut" and dysbiosis.** Dysbiosis is an overabundance of bad germs living in your gastrointestinal tract. This can be induced by medications and/or a poor diet. It can cause overeating, water weight gain and an emotional addiction to foods. Common offenders, that aggravate this problem, are dairy, wheat, chocolate and sugar.
- **Keep your thyroid healthy** – Taking a multivitamin with at least 150 mcg of iodine per day for your entire life is good insurance to prevent becoming hypothyroid. You cannot make thyroid hormone without iodine and other essential nutrients.
- **Manage your stress** – Stress often causes unconscious eating of poor vitality foods because your life has higher priorities. Stress triggers cortisol, which aggravates insulin resistance. Eating better and taking nutrients to support your adrenals during times of stress, will help you cope.
- **Improve your digestion and absorption** – Inadequate digestive enzymes or drinking ice-cold beverages inhibits digestion. Avoid drinking with meals or use room temperature or hot beverages. Use enzymes if bloating or gas is common after meals.
- **Do not skip meals** – The body thinks it is starving and actually conserves fat. You need to train your body to metabolize energy from regular meal consumption. Do not fall in the trap of substituting a caffeine beverage for a meal to stimulate your body. Again, stimulation is not energy and is a very dangerous, depleting habit.

Obesity can be the result of a period in your life when you fed yourself without conscious awareness of the consequences of your food choices. This could have been because you were simply eating similar foods as your friends or family. Or perhaps, you were living or working in an environment where healthy foods were difficult to acquire. It may also have happened because you were undergoing a long period of excessive stress, where thinking about meal planning was a very low priority.

Understand that you are choosing lifetime, dietary practices of selecting foods, beverages and activities that enhance your energy and vitality. The more you decrease or eliminate those foods and beverages that detract from your health, the greater the benefits. This does not mean you can never have ice cream or birthday cake. You will choose "party foods" only when there is an actual party. Let's not pretend there is a party every day!

Recognize the importance of exercise in your daily life to help manage your weight. A study of obese women who were unable to lose weight involved putting them on a thirty-minute daily walking program with no changes in diet. At the end of the year, the average weight loss was twenty-four lbs.

Weight training helps burn fat, not just during the exercise, but twenty-four hours per day! The most successful fat reduction comes from weight training every other day, alternating with an aerobic activity three times per week. You can take a break on the seventh day.

A TEST FOR FATTY ACIDS

If you have a health condition related to trans fatty acids, you may want to have a blood test to find out how it can be remedied. Some of the disorders of fatty acid metabolism may be due to inadequate enzyme conversions that can often be helped by nutritional supplementation.

Great Smokies Diagnostic Lab offers a blood test called the **Essential and Metabolic Fatty Acids Analysis**. It measures levels of omega-6, omega-3, omega-9 and trans fats. This test shows where your fat metabolism is disrupted, and helps your doctor choose the proper treatment. For more information on this test visit **www.gsdl.com**, or call **Great Smokies** for a doctor near you at (800) 522-4762.

> "Women with body image or eating disorders are not a special category,
> just more extreme in their response
> to a culture that emphasizes thinness
> and impossible standards of appearance for women
> instead of individuality and health."
> — Gloria Steinem

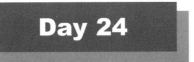

Day 24

The 4R™ Program
Remove-Replace-Reinoculate-Repair

By now, you may have noticed I put a significant amount of attention on the gastrointestinal function of my clients. It is the most common denominator that comes up in the symptoms and history of those suffering from fatigue and/or ill health. Gastrointestinal health affects energy, immune function, the brain and nervous system, the liver and kidneys, reproductive health, endocrine function and cardiovascular health.

Normalizing GI function is essential to achieving better health, energy and vitality. The **4R™ Program** was developed by **Jeffrey Bland, Ph.D.**, of **HealthComm International, Inc**. It has been thoroughly tested on thousands of clients at **The Institute for Functional Medicine™, Inc**. The 4R Program is the health regime that has produced the most significant benefit for my autoimmune disease and the various health problems of my clients.

This program supports the integrity and optimal function of the gastrointestinal lining so it can properly absorb nutrients while acting as a barrier that prevents the absorption of unwanted molecules. When this barrier has been compromised it is known as increased intestinal permeability or "leaky gut syndrome." The distance between the lining of the intestinal tract and the general circulation is only three millimeters in the healthiest of individuals. This fragile barrier can easily be altered by stress, diseases, toxic exposure, developmental age, a poor diet of medications and alcohol.

This is why the introduction of solid foods in infants must be done slowly and with a deliberate pattern. An excellent book on the subject is *Infant Nutrition*, by **Dr**. **Mark Percival** (available at **www.vitalitydoctor.com**). The popular notion in the 1950's, to give cereal to newborns (as young as two weeks of age) so they would sleep through the night, condemned many of us to an entire lifetime of severe allergies.

The consequences of increased intestinal permeability are numerous and potentially very serious. This problem does not just produce a localized effect to a single organ. It creates multiple imbalances in which function of the entire body is compromised. Altered permeability links intestinal dysfunction with problems in the brain and nervous system, hormones, skin, muscles, joints, and the immune system. Addressing problems of dysbiosis and increased intestinal permeability has allowed my patients to achieve greater energy and vitality. It is extremely gratifying when they achieve a reversal or decrease in severity of their chronic diseases.

The following tables show the symptoms and diseases associated with intestinal permeability dysfunction.

SYMPTOMS ASSOCIATED WITH INCREASED INTESTINAL PERMEABILITY
Clinical Nutrition: A Functional Approach. ©1999 by **The Institute for Functional Medicine™, Inc.**

• Fatigue and malaise	• Joint pains
• Muscle pains	• Fevers of unknown origin
• Food intolerances	• Abdominal pain
• Diarrhea	• Skin rashes
• Toxic feelings	• Cognitive and memory deficits
• Shortness of breath	• Poor exercise tolerance

DISEASES AND DRUGS ASSOCIATED WITH INCREASED INTESTINAL PERMEABILITY
Clinical Nutrition: A Functional Approach. ©1999 by **The Institute for Functional Medicine™, Inc.**

• Inflammatory bowel disease	• Irritable Bowel Syndrome
• Infectious diarrhea	• Chronic Fatigue Syndrome
• Spinal arthritis and joint pains	• NSAIDS (pain relievers)
• Acne	• Alcoholism
• Eczema	• Cytotoxic drugs
• Psoriasis	• Celiac disease
• Hives	• Dermatitis herpetiformis
• Pancreatic Insufficiency	• Autism
• Liver Dysfunction	• AIDS, HIV infection in general
• Childhood Hyperactivity	• Multiple food and chemical sensitivities

The 4R™ Program refers to the four clinical steps to intestinal rehabilitation – ***remove, replace, reinoculate*** and ***repair.*** These steps are outlined below:

REMOVE

1. "Remove" refers to the elimination of any pathogenic bacteria, fungi or parasites from the gastrointestinal tract. The bacteria and fungi can be identified by a stool culture via the **Comprehensive Digestive Stool Analysis (CDSA)**. Parasites are found by adding a three-day **Comprehensive Parasitology Analysis** to the **CDSA**.

2. This includes removing foods or toxins from the diet, to which an individual is allergic, sensitive or otherwise intolerant. A "Modified Elimination Diet" is one that contains only foods to which there is a very low overall prevalence or likelihood of allergic or antigenic reactivity, for a given population. It includes poultry, lamb, fish, legumes, brown rice, millet, buckwheat, fresh vegetables, homemade soups, fresh vegetable juices, non-citrus herbal teas, water, fresh fruit (except for strawberries and citrus), nuts, seeds, and cold-pressed oils. The "Modified Elimination Diet" excludes dairy products, refined flours and gluten grains (wheat, barley, oats and rye, spelt and kamut), corn products, yeast, beef, processed meats, eggs, fruit drinks, citrus, strawberries, dried fruits, sweetened beverages, hydrogenated fats, peanuts, artificial sweeteners, caffeine, alcohol and simple sugars. Some of these foods may be reintroduced slowly once gastrointestinal integrity is restored.

TODAY'S ACTIVITY

REPLACE

For the next phase of the 4R™ Program, we need to determine which stages of digestion may be deficient. The following questions were developed by **Lyra Heller** and **Michael Katke**, ©2000. They are available to doctors as part of a twelve-part **Health Appraisal Questionnaire** from **Metagenics, Inc.** (800) 692-9400.

Section A
- ❑ Food repeats on you after you eat (burping up food)
- ❑ Excessive burping and belching of gas following meals
- ❑ Stomach spasms and cramping during or after eating
- ❑ A sensation that food just sits in your stomach, creating uncomfortable fullness, pressure and bloating during or after a meal
- ❑ Small amounts of food fill you up immediately
- ❑ Skip meals or eat erratically because you have no appetite

Section B
- ❑ Massaging under the left side of your rib cage causes pain, tenderness or soreness
- ❑ Indigestion, fullness or tension in your abdomen is delayed, occurring two to four hours after eating
- ❑ Lower abdominal discomfort is relieved by passing gas or with a bowel movement
- ❑ Specific foods/beverages aggravate indigestion
- ❑ The consistency/form of your stool changes (e.g., from narrow to loose) within the course of a day
- ❑ Stool odor is embarassing
- ❑ Undigested food in your stool
- ❑ Three or more large bowel movements daily
- ❑ Diarrhea (frequent loose, watery stool)

Section C
- ❑ Pain or tenderness under the rib cage on the right side
- ❑ Pain at night that may move to your back or right shoulder
- ❑ Bitter fluid repeats after eating
- ❑ Feel abdominal discomfort or nausea when eating rich, fatty or fried foods
- ❑ Stool color alternates from clay colored to normal brown

REPLACE

Replace refers to the replacement of digestive factors and/or enzymes whose intrinsic, functional secretion may be limited or inadequate. The previous questions can be used in combination with the **CDSA** to determine deficiency of the various digestive factors. The **CDSA** measures several parameters of digestion and absorption.

1. Hydrochloric acid, intrinsic factor, and pepsin may be deficient if you have symptoms checked in Section A of the activity.
2. Pancreatic enzymes and proteases, lipases, amylases, cellulases and saccharidases secreted by cells lining the intestine may be deficient if you have symptoms checked in Section B.
3. Bile (fat emulsification) may be deficient if you have symptoms checked in section C.
4. Fiber may be deficient if you have small, hard, or thin diameter stools. The **CDSA** shows a need for fiber when the short-chain fatty acids (SCFA) and n-butyrate levels are low.

Consult a knowledgeable physician to help you choose the best digestive enzymes. Hydrochloric acid supplementation can aggravate gastric irritation or ulcers. A wide variety of pancreatic enzymes are available. Plant-based enzymes are generally very safe to use but may not always be the most effective. ***Day 12--Feeling Pooped?*** discussed the criteria I use for choosing a fiber supplement.

REINOCULATE

Reinoculation refers to the reintroduction of desirable gastrointestinal "friendly bacteria" (probiotics) to obtain a more desirable balance of microflora. This may include one or more of the following:

1. *Lactobacillus (acidophilus, bulgaricus, thermophilus)*
2. *Bifidobacteria (bifidus, infantis, longum, breve)*
3. *Saccaromyces boulardi*
4. The addition of fructooligosaccharides (FOS) or inulin (a carbohydrate) to the diet has been shown to selectively support the growth and sustain the presence of these desirable micro-flora, especially *Bifidobacteria.*

REPAIR

Repair refers to providing direct nutritional support for regeneration and healing of the gastrointestinal cell wall structure and function. The GI mucosal cells represent the largest mass of rapidly growing and reproducing cells in the bodies of normal individuals. The most critical nutritional factors include antioxidants such as vitamins C, E, A and beta-carotene, the minerals zinc and manganese, the amino acids cysteine, N-acetylcysteine and glutamine, the tripeptide glutathione and the carbohydrate inulin and/or FOS.

Metagenics makes two products for the repair of the gastrointestinal cells. The first is a medical food developed by **Dr. Jeffrey Bland** called **UltraClear SUSTAIN®**. This product is a rice-based formula that contains everything previously mentioned, and more. **UltraClear SUSTAIN®** contains five hundred milligrams of glutamine per serving.

Metagenics introduced another product, **Glutagenics™**, in March of 2000, which contains a much higher dose of L-glutamine (3,500 mg. per teaspoon), along with deglycyrrhized licorice root and aloe leaf extract. The licorice root has the glycyrrhizin removed to avoid side effects for people who have high blood pressure. Research has shown that as much as ten to twenty grams of glutamine per day are needed to repair the intestinal wall.

Glutamine is the most abundant amino acid found in muscle. It plays a role in muscle recovery and prevents muscle breakdown. More research is needed to determine whether glutamine improves the intestinal muscular contractions known as peristalsis. A few years ago, before I was aware of the function of glutamine, I saw a few patients with a severe lack of intestinal peristalsis. These patients had been dependent on enemas and colon hydro-therapy, but they may have just been severely deficient in glutamine.

The 4R™ Program is important for healing conditions associated with increased intestinal permeability, any overt GI diseases and certainly intestinal cancers. From the discussions I have had with clients, this avenue of healing is unknown or not utilized. Since prevention is far more desirable than intestinal surgery, it is my hope that this extremely valuable program becomes more widely known.

For physicians interested in more training on the 4R™ Program, contact the **Institute for Functional Medicine**, at **www.fxmed.com** or (800) 228-0622.

> "You don't develop courage by being happy in your relationships everyday.
> You develop it by surviving difficult times and challenging adversity."
> — Barbara DeAngelis

3 DAY FOOD & ACTIVITY DIARY

	Date:	Date:	Date:
Morning Meal Time:			
Snack			
Noon Meal Time:			
Snack			
Evening Meal Time:			
Snack			
Symptoms (Physical & Emotional)			
Exercise Type & Duration			

Day 25

"Anger is the most impotent of passions.
It affects nothing it goes about,
and hurts the one who is possessed by it
more than the one against whom it is directed."
— Clarendon

Love Your Liver

The liver is, by far, the most important detoxification organ of our body. The liver is literally the organ that *lets you live.* When the liver is impacted by serious disease or cancer, it causes tremendous fatigue and a decrease in quality of life. Many people suffer from a "congested" or "sluggish" liver that is becoming less efficient at detoxification. This can progress into more serious problems, especially if the liver is suddenly faced with increased demands for detoxification such as from alcohol, a medication or an exposure to chemicals such as pesticides.

When you understand how to keep the liver healthy you can greatly improve your energy, vitality and longevity. Proper liver function is imperative for preventing cancer anywhere in the body. This chapter will explore the many detoxification reactions that occur in the liver and how to keep them running efficiently with proper nutritional support.

In Oriental medicine, the liver and gall bladder are the organs associated with anger. Considering the increase in road rage and other abusive behaviors, these organs need some attention. A poorly functioning liver or gall bladder can make you irritable but it works both ways. A person who has gotten into a pattern of excessive anger and rage will eventually create disease in their liver and gallbladder.

The irritability associated with PMS and menopause, can often be very easily be alleviated by improving liver function. If a person genuinely wants to decrease their irritability, they need to avoid substances that irritate the liver and gall bladder. Some examples would be alcohol, deep-fried foods, caffeine, chocolate and other hydrogenated fats, and excessive use of medications, especially over-the-counter pain relievers.

Many people think they can take unlimited quantities of pain relievers because they are available without prescription. This is a very dangerous habit that not only stresses the liver but also depletes your body's ability to make its own pain relievers. The cause of pain should always be investigated. As a chiropractor, I have seen many patients who took daily doses of pain relievers for months or years before they sought chiropractic care and received more permanent relief.

DIAGNOSING LIVER DYSFUNCTION

A simple, Oriental method for identifying liver malfunction is to observe the side edges of your tongue. If your liver is not detoxifying adequately, your tongue will enlarge and push up against your teeth. The outline of your teeth causes a scalloped indentation along the sides of the tongue, much like the edges of a piecrust. Geographic tongue, which is seen as colored blotches on the tongue that look like a map, is also associated with liver dysfunction. An Oriental diagnostic sign of liver dysfunction on the face is the appearance of deep vertical lines between the eyebrows.

When the gall bladder is malfunctioning, from gallstones or inflammation, you will sometimes have pain at the front, lower edge of your right rib cage. The liver does not have any pain fibers so it cannot signal its dysfunction in that way. Sometimes, liver/gall bladder problems cause pain in the right shoulder, shoulder blade or between the shoulder blades. You may also develop abdominal discomfort or nausea after eating rich, fatty or fried foods.

Frequently, having blood work done to look for the cause of fatigue is the first awareness of a liver problem. When liver function tests show elevated bilirubin, SGOT (aka AST), alkaline phosphatase, SGPT (aka ALT), GGTP, LDH, etc., this indicates that cellular damage is occurring in the liver. An elevation of total cholesterol is an early sign the liver is having difficulty metabolizing fats.

TODAY'S ACTIVITY

Feel the rib cage area just below the right side of your chest. See if there are any tender areas on the top surface or just under the edge of the rib cage.

Examine your tongue in the mirror to see if you have the scalloped edges or discolorations mentioned above. Take a look at your Food and Activity Diaries to see if you have listed any days of feeling irritable. Check to see what you have been consuming in the few days prior to that. Look for excessive fried foods, pizza, alcohol, chocolate, artificial sweeteners and preservatives, rich desserts or foods with hydrogenated fats.

Add foods to your diet that improve detoxification such as kale or collards and salads. Observe whether your grumpiness subsides.

LIVER FUNCTION

The liver is a complex organ that plays an important role in energy metabolism and detoxification. It has to neutralize a wide range of toxic chemicals, both from the environment and those produced internally. The liver's ability to detoxify efficiently is compromised greatly by nutritional depletion. We have discussed at length how the quality of food and beverages affects our intestinal tract. The excess liquid from the digestive contents is absorbed directly to the liver by numerous veins along the colon. A toxic bowel causes tremendous burden on the liver.

Measurements of our fat tissues for chemicals reveals that nearly everyone has ingested and stored various herbicides and pesticides such as DDT, dioxin, PCB and PCP. Even organic foods contain naturally occuring toxic products that require effective detoxification.

Proper functioning of the liver's detoxification systems is especially important for the prevention of cancer. Up to ninety percent of all cancers are thought to be due to the effects of exposure to carcinogens combined with deficiencies of the nutrients needed for proper functioning of the detoxification and immune systems. High levels of exposure to carcinogens, combined with slow or impaired detoxification enzymes, significantly increases overall suceptibility to cancer. A study of chemical plant workers from Turin, Italy, who had unusally high rates of bladder cancer, showed a correlation with liver activity. Measurement of liver detoxification enzymes showed abnormal function in those who developed cancer.

THREE MAJOR DETOXIFICATION FUNCTIONS OF THE LIVER

I. One of the liver's primary functions is to filter our blood. Almost two quarts of blood per minute pass through the liver for detoxification. When the liver is damaged, such as with alcoholism or hepatitis, significant numbers of bacteria from the colon and other toxins pass on through, unable to be neutralized.

II. Another method of liver detoxification involves the synthesis and secretion of bile. Each day, our livers manufacture about one quart of bile, which serves as a carrier to dump many toxic substances into our intestines. If we have adequate fiber in our intestines, these toxins will be absorbed by the fiber and excreted. If not, we will *reabsorb* the toxins.

If the excretion of bile is inhibited, toxins will stay in the liver longer. This is known as cholestasis and has several causes. The most common cause is gallstones or bile that is too thick and viscous. Nutrients that improve methylation (described under Phase II Liver Detoxification function) will help this condition.

Alcohol ingestion is another common cause of cholestasis. As little as one ounce of alcohol can produce damage to the liver in sensitive individuals. Alcohol damage shows up as fatty infiltration of the liver and an increase in size. Other causes of cholestasis include:

- Endotoxins (toxins produced internally)
- Hereditary disorders (Gilbert's syndrome)
- Hyperthyroidism or thyroxine drugs
- Viral hepatitis
- Pregnancy
- Certain drugs or chemicals:
  - Natural and synthetic steroidal hormones – anabolic steroids, estrogens, birth control pills
  - Aminosalicylic acid
  - Chlorothiazide
  - Erythromycin estolate
  - Mepazine
  - Phenylbutazone
  - Sulphadiazine
  - Thiouracil

III. The third method of detoxification, in which unwanted chemicals and toxins are neutralized, involves a two-step enzymatic process, known as Phase I and Phase II. This is how we neutralize and metabolize caffeine, alcohol, drugs, pesticides, colon toxins, hormones and inflammatory chemicals such as histamine.

Phase I detoxification involves a group of fifty to one hundred enzymes, known collectively as cytochrome P450. Phase I enzymes directly neutralize some chemicals, but most are converted to intermediate forms that need to be processed by Phase II enzymes. The intermediate forms are more chemically active and are therefore more toxic than the original chemical. If we are metabolizing a lot of substances that drive Phase I detoxification, it is imperative that there be enough nutrients in Phase II to neutralize these dangerous toxins.

This is why some people go into acute liver or kidney failure from taking over-the-counter medications such as acetaminophen or ibuprofen. I know a young man who went into acute kidney failure from just a single dose of ibuprofen, even though he had taken the same drug with no ill effects just two weeks prior. When I inquired about his dietary habits, he had been drinking about eight cups of coffee daily, which causes a lot of Phase I activity. His Phase II nutrients finally got depleted (he was not taking any vitamins) and the intermediate form of ibuprofen was unable to be neutralized.

The main job of Phase II detoxification is to make toxins water-soluble to allow them to be excreted safely by the kidneys. This is also related to why the Italian chemical workers previously mentioned, ended up with bladder cancer. The free radical damage of these chemicals going through the kidneys and being stored in the bladder contribtued to the cancer.

There has been a lot of concern in recent years about a medical condition known as "overactive bladder." Perhaps, the bladder is overactive because of improperly detoxified chemicals harassing it. We should consider improving liver function in such patients rather than squelching the message of a traumatized organ.

SYMPTOMS OF PHASE I DEFICIENCY

People with underactive Phase I enzymes will experience caffeine sensitivity, intolerance to perfumes and other environmental chemicals, and an increased risk of liver disease. The nutrients needed by Phase I detoxification enzymes include copper, magnesium, zinc, vitamin C, flavonoids, vitamins B2, B3, B6, B12, folic acid, and glutathione. Magnesium deficiency substantially increases the toxicity of many drugs.

Intolerance to odors and a reaction to sulfur-containing foods and drugs is also specifically related to a deficiency of the trace mineral, molybdenum. This includes the sulfite allergy caused by eating from salad bars. All of these nutrients are found in a good quality multivitamin/mineral, such as **Multigenics®** by **Metagenics**.

Recent research shows the cytochrome P450 enzymes are also found in other parts of the body, especially in brain cells. Inadequate levels of antioxidants and nutrients in the brain result in increased rate of damage to nerve cells, which is seen in Alzheimer's and Parkinson's disease patients.

FOODS FOR DETOXIFICATION

The Brassica family of vegetables, i.e., cabbage, broccoli, and Brussels sprouts, contain chemical compounds that stimulate both Phase I and Phase II detoxification enzymes. They contain a powerful anti-cancer compound (indole-3-carbinol), which is also a stimulant of detoxifying enzymes in the gut.

Oranges, tangerines and the seeds of caraway and dill contain limonene, a phytochemical that strongly induces both Phase I and Phase II detoxification enzymes that neutralize carcinogens.

On the other hand, eight ounces of grapefruit juice contains a flavonoid called naringenin that can *decrease* cytochrome P450 activity by thirty percent. This can cause substantial problems because it decreases the rate of elimination of drugs from the blood and has been found to alter their clinical activity and toxicity.

Curcumin, the yellow compound in turmeric, inhibits Phase I while stimulating Phase II. This can be very useful in preventing certain types of cancer. Curcumin has been found to inhibit carcinogens, such as benzpyrene (found in charcoal-broiled meat). Curcumin has also been shown to directly inhibit the growth of cancer cells.

Phase I enzyme activity decreases in old age. When you combine that with lack of exercise and poor nutrition, the elderly have significant impairment of detoxification capacity. This explains why toxic reactions to medications, especially within those taking multiple drugs, are seen so commonly in the elderly.

DRUGS AND ENVIRONMENTAL TOXINS THAT INCREASE PHASE I ACTIVITY INCLUDE:

Drugs:
- Alcohol
- Caffeine
- Nicotine
- Phenobarbital
- Sulfonamides
- Steroids

Environmental Toxins:
- Carbon tetrachloride
- Exhaust fumes
- Paint fumes
- Dioxin
- Pesticides

DRUGS AND BOTANICALS THAT INHIBIT PHASE I DETOXIFICATION INCLUDE:

- Benzodiazepines (e.g., Halcion, Centrax, Librium, Valium, etc.)
- Antihistamines (used for allergies)
- Cimetidine and other stomach-acid secretion blocking drugs (used for acid reflux)
- Ketoconozole (the anti-fungal drug, Diflucan)
- Sulphaphenazole
- Curcumin, capsaicin, eugenol and calendula

PHASE II DETOXIFICATION

This phase of detoxification involves biochemical reactions that either neutralize the toxin or make it more easily excreted in the urine or bile. There are six Phase II detoxification pathways: glutathione conjugation, amino acid conjugation, methylation, sulfation, acetylation and glucuronidation.

I know this sounds complex. What you need to know is these processes require important nutritional factors to drive them. The majority of these nutrients are found in a good diet and the "Big 3" nutritional supplements that were mentioned in *Day 2*. The antioxidant formula, especially, has many of the nutrients mentioned for liver detoxification. The whey protein concentrate mentioned in the protein chapter is also an important source of several amino acids needed for these processes.

THESE PHASE II DETOXIFICATION PATHWAYS ARE NEEDED TO DETOXIFY THE FOLLOWING SUBSTANCES:

- **Glutathione conjugation:** acetominophen, nicotine, insecticides, carcinogens
- **Amino acid conjugation:** benzoate, aspirin
- **Methylation:** dopamine, epinephrine, histamine, thiouracil
- **Sulfation:** aniline dyes, coumarin, acetominophen, methyl-dopa, estrogen, testosterone, thyroid hormone
- **Acetylation:** sulfonamides, mescaline
- **Glucuronidation:** acetominophen, morphine, diazepam, digitalis, aspirin, vanillin, benzoates

---

THE IMPORTANT NUTRIENTS AND FOODS NEEDED FOR THESE PROCESSES INCLUDE:

- **Glutathione conjugation:** Glutathione, vitamin B6, Brassica family foods
- **Amino acid conjugation:** Glycine, adequate protein
- **Methylation:** S-adenosylmethionine (SAM)– from choline, methionine, betaine, folic acid and vitamin B12
- **Sulfation:** Cysteine, methionine, molybdenum, taurine
- **Acetylation:** Acetyl-CoA (from energy metabolism), vitamins B1, B5 and C
- **Glucuronication:** Glucuronic acid, fish oils, limonene-containing foods

---

CLINICAL INDICATORS OF PROBABLE PHASE II DYSFUNCTION:

- **Glutathione conjugation:** Chronic exposure to chemical toxins, chronic alcohol consumption
- **Amino acid conjugation:** Intestinal toxicity, toxemia of pregnancy
- **Methylation:** PMS, estrogen excess, gall bladder dysfunction, oral contraceptive use
- **Sulfation:** Intestinal toxicity, Parkinson's disease, Alzheimer's disease, rheumatoid arthritis
- **Acetylation:** Unknown
- **Glucuronidation:** Gilbert's disease, yellow discoloration of eyes and skin, not due to hepatitis

One way to make use of these charts is to make sure you are getting the nutrients listed, especially if you have a related condition. SAM-e is a recently introduced nutritional product that improves methylation. However, it is a fairly unstable and expensive product. It is more cost-effective to supplement with the lipotrophic (fat-metabolizing) factors – methionine, choline, and betaine, that help the body make SAM.

Metagenics makes a product called **Lipo-Gen™**, which provides all of these nutrients (plus others) to help with fat metabolism. I have used this product for many years to help people with gall bladder problems, high cholesterol and the irritable type of PMS. Deficient methylation has also recently been associated with heart disease, cancer and Alzheimer's disease.

SILYMARIN

The herb *Silibum marianum* (milk thistle,) aka silymarin, has been shown to protect the liver as well as enhance the detoxification processes. Silymarin protects the liver through several important mechanisms: acting as a powerful antioxidant, increasing glutathione synthesis, and increasing the rate of liver tissue regeneration. The antioxidant activity of silymarin is many times more potent than vitamins E and C. Silymarin prevents the depletion of glutathione and can increase the level of glutathione in the liver by up to thirty-five percent. **Metagenics** has a product called **Silymarin 80**. It is a seventy milligram milk thistle seed extract tablet, standardized to eighty percent.

FASTING FOR DETOXIFICATION

Fasting has been used as a detoxification method to increase the elimination of wastes and enhance the healing processes of the body. People are most familiar with fasting as the total abstinence from anything but water for a certain period of time. However, because many people who need fasting are also depleted of many nutrients that support detoxification, it is wiser to choose a more moderate approach. Modified fasting can be a day with just a variety of fresh vegetable juices or an entire day of only raw foods. The type of fasting I most frequently recommend is a combination of medical foods for detoxification used with vegetable juices and a restricted list of low allergy potential foods. The "Modified Elimination Diet" was described in *Day 24 – The 4R™ Program*. This type of detoxification program can be continued for a month or more.

Dr. Jeffrey Bland has developed two patented medical foods, distributed by **Metagenics**, that enhance liver detoxification. **UltraClear®**, supports both Phase I and Phase II detoxification. **UltraClear PLUS®,** was developed for those individuals who have uneven activity between Phase I detoxification and Phase II detoxification. It more heavily supports Phase II detoxification. They both use a pleasant-tasting, low-allergy-potential rice protein concentrate. They often need to be introduced slowly in combination with the "Modified Elimination Diet," and are best used under the guidance of a holistic physician.

Metagenics also has a phytonutrient supplement that helps support Phase II enzyme activity. It contains broccoli powder, quercetin, garlic bulb powder, turmeric and limonene. That product is called **PhytoPhase®**.

As you can see from this chapter, the liver is one of our most complex organs and demands a wide variety of nutrients to operate efficiently. When it lacks those nutrients, the health of the entire body is in danger of developing cancer and many serious degenerative illnesses. All of this dysfunction accumulates in small increments with problems that often have no symptoms until they become severe.

We cannot underestimate the stress of medications to the liver. Adverse Drug Reactions have been in the top ten causes of death for several years now. The most recent figure in 1997 listed them as the fifth leading cause of death. There are presently more deaths annually related to the pain relievers known as Non-Steroidal AntiInflammatory Drugs (NSAID's) than AIDS-related deaths. We have to take good care of our livers to be able to better handle the many important functions we demand of it. If your liver could talk, it would tell you, "Feed me well and take your vitamins!"

> Always use the word impossible with the greatest caution."
> — Werner von Braun

Day 26

"It is not because things are difficult that we do not dare,
it is because we do not dare that they are difficult."

—Seneca

Detoxification & Colon Cleansing

All people have toxic substances in their bodies. The sources of these toxins are external pollutants, the ingestion of chemicals in our food and beverages and toxins that are made within the body itself (endotoxins). The key steps to decreasing your body's toxic burden are avoidance, supplementation to enhance detoxification, and colon cleansing.

We have already discussed ways to avoid toxin exposure and nutritional supplementation that will encourage the body's ability to detoxify. When a person has not been taking nutritional supplements, they often have very sluggish detoxification abilities. Sometimes, people have to start a supplementation program very slowly to make sure all of the avenues of elimination are ready to do their job.

This is where colon cleansing comes in. If you are constipated, you will not be able to detoxify properly and can even temporarily feel worse. You may also experience a "die-off" reaction as you take medications or natural remedies that kill yeasts and other germs. If you know how to prevent these symptoms, you can avoid the majority of problems.

These symptoms are referred to as a "detoxification response." They can include increased fatigue, cold or flu-like symptoms, muscle or joint pains, headaches, nausea, diarrhea, constipation, fever, rashes or the discharge of increased mucus from the nose or respiratory passages. To minimize or prevent these symptoms you can take the following steps:

1. Decrease the dosage on your new supplements.
2. Try to decrease the rate at which you work on eliminating harmful dietary habits such as caffeine, chocolate, sugar, artificial sweeteners, etc. Caffeine is especially notorious for causing withdrawal headaches.
3. Increase the number of enzymes you are taking. In addition to the enzymes you are taking to digest your meals, you can take some of the plant-based enzymes between meals. For instance, bromelain (a pineapple enzyme) is great to use at bedtime and in the morning to digest excessive mucus and decrease inflammation. I have also used **SpectraZyme®,** from **Metagenics**, both with and between meals, for decreasing a variety of toxicity symptoms.
4. Drink plenty of pure water, herb teas and vegetable juices.
5. Avoid heavy foods such as dairy, fried foods and large portions of meat. Avoid sweets and starches such as bread, bagels, pasta, cereal, crackers, cookies and pastry.

6. Engage in light exercise such as walking ten to fifteen minutes, once or twice daily.

7. Do ten minutes of breathing exercises.

8. Get plenty of rest.

9. If the bowels are not moving well, consider doing some form of colon cleansing. Instructions for colon cleansing will follow in this chapter. Fiber and probiotics (intestinal bacterial products) might also be considered to improve bowel function.

Beginning in the 1880's, much attention was paid to the relationship between maldigestion and much of the chronic illness seen in patients. "Death Begins in the Colon" was the warning of early doctors who warned that sluggish bowel function can cause a toxemia that has far-reaching consequences to nearly every part of the body. In the first fifty years of the 1900's, children and adults took doses of castor oil and did enemas to induce better bowel cleansing. As it turns out, we now know castor oil is very good at suppressing several species of yeast in our bowel.

In the second half of the 1900's, modern doctors got away from being concerned with the colon function and relegated the treatment of diarrhea and constipation to the over-the-counter section of the pharmacy. Patients were essentially expected to figure it out themselves and only consult with doctors when they had major problems that became severe or unmanageable.

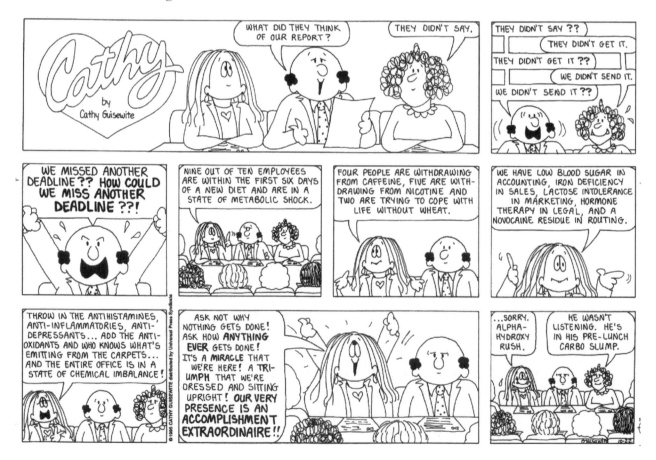

When doctors stopped inquiring about colon function, patients became too embarrassed to discuss the topic and began forming their own varying opinions about what was normal function. Recently, I asked a patient if she was experiencing constipation or diarrhea and she replied that she was not. I learned long ago to never stop at that one question. My next question was to inquire how frequently she had a bowel movement and she replied, "Every three days."

Often when I start asking my patients details about their bowel activity, I can tell this is the first time they have had this type of conversation with a doctor. Discussing the characteristics of normal and abnormal intestinal function listed in *Day 11--Feeling Pooped?* often sheds light on some of the causes of their health problems. Having a greater awareness of what abnormal symptoms mean and how they can be corrected prevents small problems from turning into major diseases.

There is probably not a single person in America who has not expereinced the whole range of bowel function, from constipation to diarrhea, at some point in their life. Monitoring colon function is one way to keep tabs on the health of your entire body. The whole digestive system is one part of your body that gives you the most feedback on your diet and lifestyle. We must track down the cause rather than getting temporary relief with medications such as antacids, laxatives and diarrhea remedies.

Dysbiosis, as described in *Day 13--What's Bugging You*, is a state of living with harmful intestinal flora. These organisms create a low-grade infection that induces disease by altering the nutrition or immune function of their host. Dysbiosis may result in processes opposite those found in a healthy gut. For instance, they may degrade vitamins rather than synthesize them. They may suppress immune function rather than enhance it. Slowly but surely, these abnormal organisms begin to erode our health.

Most importantly, dysbiosis may impair digestion and detoxification. This can result in the persistence of certain hormones and drugs and the formation of carcinogens, including estrogen-related cancers. This may also account for some cases of premenstrual syndrome, as deficient bowel flora has been noted in PMS patients.

HEALTH BEGINS IN THE COLON!

We cannot ignore this important organ. It is intimately associated with our wellness, energy and vitality. Achieving more normal bowel function is *mandatory* for good health. This is why I have devoted four chapters of this book to understanding intestinal function.

Today we are going to learn about the anatomy and function of the colon (see Figure 26.1). The colon, or large intestine, starts down in the lower right quadrant of your abdomen where your appendix is located. The large intestine is separated from the small intestine by a one-way valve known as the ileo-cecal valve. This name comes from the last part of the small intestine (ileum) and the first part of the colon (the cecum).

The ileo-cecal valve prevents the colon's contents from backing up into the small intestine when you become extremely constipated. Bowel toxicity irritates the ileo-cecal valve, and may cause further damage to the small intestine. The appendix is believed to be a small immune organ that helps fight inflammation in this area.

From the cecum, the colon travels straight upward toward the liver and is known as the ascending colon. It then makes an abrupt turn (known as the hepatic flexure) and travels across your abdomen around the level of your navel. This section is known as the transverse colon. It turns abruptly again on the left side of the abdomen under the spleen, known as the splenic flexure. It then heads down to the rectum, which is the last few inches before the anus.

This last section follows the previous naming pattern and is known as the descending colon. The lower part of the descending colon is also known as the Sigmoid colon. When you have a Sigmoidoscope exam, it only examines as far as the splenic flexure, which is why it is not considered as valuable a test for screening colon cancer as the colonoscopy. The colonoscopy examines all the way to the cecum.

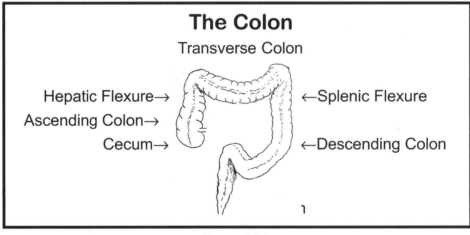

Figure 26.1

Lie down on a flat surface with your knees bent and use your finger tips to feel the various sections of the colon. Start down by the appendix, work your way up toward the liver, across your belly and then down the left side to the area where the left groin meets the pubic bone. Note if any sections feel tender. This could indicate inflammation. Feel whether the colon is soft or hard. Note if palpating this area makes you feel nauseated.

One of the main functions of the colon is to absorb various liquids from the digestive contents and excrete bowel movements in a solid mass. The entire colon has several veins attached that join together and head straight to the liver. The quality of the digestion has everything to do with whether the liquids going to the liver are neutral or toxic. When the colon's contents are extremely toxic, it spells bad news for the liver, and is a major contributing factor to liver disease.

When the colon is constipated for a long time, the waste has nowhere to go but to expand the thin walls of the colon. First, the pressure may cause outpouchings known as diverticuli. Later, the expansion may stretch the entire wall of the colon, resulting in a condition known as megacolon. This often prolapses the entire abdomen, causing a protruding gut low in the abdomen that looks like a shelf extending out from the pubic bone.

Sometimes the expansion of the colon causes a severe loss of the ability to perform the wave-like, peristalsis muscular activity that causes normal bowel activity. For these individuals, different forms of colon cleansing might be considered.

There are two basic categories of colon cleansing. The first is from the "top down" and the second is from the "bottom up" (colon hydrotherapy). The typical method of dealing with constipation is laxatives, which work by irritating the bowel to expel its contents. This can have a weakening effect on the bowel and create dependency. A good "top down" colon cleanser should be mostly concerned with increasing mechanical action to clean the colon.

INTESTINAL CLEANSING PRODUCTS

V. E. Irons was a man who became a student of health at the age of forty, when he was stricken with an arthritis called Ankylosing Spondylitis. We now know that this arthritis has a strong correlation to the colon and is associeted with the presence of an intestinal germ known as ***Klebsiella pneumoniae***. **Mr. Irons** developed a colon-cleansing program in 1953 that is still very much in use today. **Mr. Irons'** health was restored and he began a second family at the age of seventy-two and fathered his last child at the age of eighty. He passed away in 1993 at the age of ninety-eight.

The **V.E. Irons** colon program has a very strong mechanical action for cleansing the colon. These products should be used under the supervision of a holistic health care provider who is familiar with their action. Contact **Springreen Products, Inc.,** at (800) 544-8147, to find a professional who can help you with this type of cleansing.

V.E. Irons formulas include ample amounts of montmorillonite, a derivative of bentonite clay that is excellent for latching onto toxins. The formula uses psyllium as a fiber to enhance bowel activity to carry the toxins out of the body. These two products are also valuable for cleansing heavy metals and during amalgam filling removal.

The **V.E. Irons Seven Day Cleansing Program** also utilizes other enzymes and green products to assist the body in detoxification. Many health practitioners recommend doing a cleansing program at least four times per year, as the seasons change.

Day 24--The 4-R™ Program, is the primary program I use with my patients. It involves a comprehensive program of intestinal rehabilitation that is a more permanent solution to digestive problems. Colon cleansing methods are just one phase of the 4R™ Program--Remove.

COLON CLEANSING

The two main forms of colon cleansing are enemas and colon hydrotherapy (usually performed by a therapist). Enemas have been used since ancient Egypt in the fourteenth century B.C. In the seventeenth century of Paris Society, it was an acceptable practice to have as many as three or four enemas per day with the belief that this was essential to well being.

There are times when I am working with people with severe toxicity issues that these forms of colon cleansing can be useful. When a person is trying to improve their organs of detoxification or kill bad germs in the gut, their colon function has to be adequate or else they will feel overwhelmed by their body's detoxification attempts. Symptoms are caused when you reabsorb the toxins because of inadequate bowel function to expel them.

To avoid "detoxification response" symptoms such as headaches, nausea, muscle aches, etc., you should consider short-term methods of colon cleansing. Performing a warm-water enema at home can be a fast remedy to such symptoms. It is not necessary to buy a medicinal enema preparation from the pharmacy. Warm water is adequate for loosening waste.

Please Note: Enemas should only be performed with the advice of your physician when you are pregnant, suffer from hypertension or congestive heart disease, have diarrhea or bloody stools, suspect colon cancer, have had prior colon surgery or have recently had any type of surgery.

ENEMA INSTRUCTIONS

Enema bags can be purchased in any pharmacy and are often made so they can double as a hot water bottle. I usually recommend an enema be performed in a bathtub with a shallow amount of warm water to be more comfortable. This way, if any leakage occurs, it is much easier to clean a bathtub than the bathroom floor.

The enema bag comes with a long tube and a plastic applicator that will be easily inserted a couple of inches into the rectum with a lubricating gel. The enema bag should be fitted with the tubing and applicator and then filled with warm water (filtered is preferable). Crimp the tubing to prevent water from coming out of the applicator as you hang the bag on the showerhead with the plastic or metal hook provided.

Put the gel on the applicator and then lie down on your left side in the bathtub with your knees bent. Bend the right knee forward to be able to insert the tip gently into the rectum. Continue crimping the tube but allow small amounts of water to enter the colon. If you feel pressure stop the inflow of water until it passes. If the pressure is not relieved, remove the tube and go to the toilet to evacuate. Wait on the toilet for about five minutes so you can be sure you will not have to go again immediately. Do not be concerned that you cannot retain the entire quart bag of water. It is a good sign to have peristalsis triggered with only part of the water inserted.

After evacuating, get back into the bath and try to finish the quart. If needed, go back to the toilet before finishing. When you finish inserting the water, lie onto your back and massage the colon gently from the descending colon upward to loosen the fecal matter. This may trigger peristalsis again, so quickly remove your applicator and get back on the toilet. You are finished except for bowel evacuation and bathtub cleanup.

COLON HYDROTHERAPY

Colon hydrotherapy is available from an estimated five thousand colon hydrotherapists in the United States. Colon hydrotherapy involves introducing filtered and temperature regulated water into the colon. The fecal matter is softened and loosened, resulting in evacuation through normal peristalsis through an outflow tube. This process is repeated several times to allow a greater degree of cleansing than can be achieved with an enema.

Be sure the practitioner you choose uses modern, FDA-registered equipment with sterile, disposable, single-use rectal tubes and speculae. The **International Association for Colon Hydrotherapy (I-ACT)** advocates the highest standards of education and professional conduct to assure properly administered colon hydrotherapy. Level One Certification involves one hundred hours of training, Level Two, five hundred hours and Level Three requires one thousand hours. For more information, you can contact I-ACT at (210) 366-2888 or by visiting their web site at **www.i-act.org**.

ACCORDING TO I-ACT, THE CONTRAINDICATIONS TO COLON HYDROTHERAPY INCLUDE:

- Uncontrolled hypertension
- Congestive heart failure
- Aneurysm
- Severe anemia
- GI hemorrhage/perforation
- Severe hemorrhoids
- Ist and 3rd trimester pregnancy
- Renal insufficiency
- Cirrhosis
- Colon cancer
- Fissures/fistulas
- Abdominal hernia
- Recent colon surgery

HOME ENEMA KITS

Another method of colon cleansing is a home device known as a **Colema Board®**, developed in 1975. This board rests between a chair and your toilet with a five-gallon water device sitting on your toilet tank. This allows a one-time insertion of the tube and continuous evacuations directly into your toilet without removal of the tip. It provides much more water than an enema in the convenience of your home. This device pays for itself very quickly when compared to visits for professional colon hydrotherapy. More information can be obtained from the web site **www.colema-boards.com** or (800) 745-2446.

Although it may seem unpleasant to utilize colon cleansing, it is a fast remedy for unpleasant symptoms of excessive toxicity. I want to emphasize again that colon cleanses should be considered for use during short periods, a few times per year. They should not be used on a regular or frequent basis. And of course, the cause of bowel dysfunction should always be investigated by a holistic physician or a gastrointestinal specialist. Your goal is to achieve healthy bowel function with diet, proper digestion, adequate fiber and good intestinal flora. A healthy colon pays big dividends with improved organ function throughout the body.

"Great changes may not happen right away, but with effort even the difficult may become easy."
— Bill Blackman

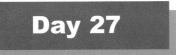

"To keep the body in good health is a duty…
otherwise we shall not be able to keep our mind strong and clear."

— Buddha

Weight Training Made Easy

One of the most important ways to make yourself feel more physically and mentally powerful and energetic is to build stronger muscles through weight training. Hopefully, by now you are starting to feel more vitality. This may be a good time to add some weight training to your life. Exercise guru, **Jack LaLanne**, who is in his mid-eighties, is a powerful testimony for growing older while remaining strong and vital to enjoy life to the fullest.

Some people drastically curtail their physical activities as they grow older and this very quickly diminishes their body's capabilities. They have a mental image of an elderly person belonging in a rocking chair instead of as an energetic person who travels or explores new activities. A recent survey in America revealed that there were still fifty thousand people in their nineties earning a paycheck.

In the "olden days," people did not have to make any special effort to gain muscle strength. Day to day life was much more physically demanding. Exercise equipment and gyms were unheard of. In our quest to spend more time at a desk accomplishing mental tasks, our muscles have become soft and weaker. This sedentary lifestyle contributes greatly to fatigue.

People of any age – with a doctor's approval – can increase their strength with a simple weight training program. Studies of frail seniors in their eighties and nineties have shown weight training can improve strength, walking ability and balance. Increasing strength is particularly important in preventing falls, which are more prevalent with elderly people. Weight training is also a valuable way to strengthen bones and prevent osteoporosis.

A recent study of men ages sixty to seventy-five, at **Ohio University,** who completed weight training exercises at eighty to eighty-five percent of their maximum, showed gains in leg muscle strength up to eighty-four percent over sixteen weeks. The scientists also found that the men who exercised gained endurance – their hearts worked less hard at a given intensity in a treadmill test. These results were published in the ***Journal of Gerontology.***

More people are using weight training to increase their metabolic rate, which in turn improves their body fat ratio. Exercise and proper nutrition are the healthiest ways to increase metabolic rate and build lean muscle mass. Hormones and "thermogenic" stimulants, such as Ma huang or ephedrine, are not worth the health risks. Steroid hormones are the dangerous muscle-bulking drugs we most commonly associate with weight training. However, human growth hormone (HGH) is another controversial drug that is becoming increasingly popular. I believe that we do not know enough about the long-term consequences of using HGH.

BODY FAT

I measure body fat percentage on each patient to help them understand how their eating habits affect their health. It is not unusual to find people of all ages, especially women, with body fat percentages as high as forty or fifty percent. The high end of normal for women over the age of thirty is twenty-seven percent. Sporting goods stores sell electronic scales that measure both weight and body fat percentage. They measure bioelectrical impedance through your bare feet without any perceived sensation.

HEALTHY BODY FAT RANGE		
	Under 30 yrs old	**Over 30 yrs old**
Male	14%-20%	17%-23%
Female	17%-24%	20%-27%

Measuring body fat can help identify a new health classification of patients known as MONW, which stands for "metabolically obese, normal weight." This patient does not look overweight but their body fat is increasing and their lean muscle mass is decreasing. As I mentioned in ***Day 5--The Sugar Blues,*** this is a strong sign of insulin dysregulation.

I also evaluate this condition further by doing grip strength tests on everyone. I have seen middle-aged men with the same grip strength as an average healthy woman. Testosterone declines when hormones, such as cortisol and insulin, are out of balance. It is amazing how much improvement in grip strength and body fat percentage can occur in just one month's time when the person changes their diet, nutrition and stress management habits. These conservative measures should be attempted before resorting to the use of hormone medications.

Another area to watch is an increased waist-to-hip ratio, the so-called "apple" body type. When the waist becomes bigger than the hips, health problems like heart disease and diabetes ultimately follow. Weight training and a proper diet are the best ways to control your waistline.

METHODS OF WEIGHT TRAINING

Weight training can be as simple as lifting soup cans, water bottles, or the more traditional dumbbells or barbells. You can even increase your lower body workout by holding dumbbells when you do deep knee bends or lunges. Try using ankle weights while doing leg lifts to the front, side and back. To avoid injuries it is best to warm up first with at least ten minutes of aerobic activity.

Do not skip the warmup step!

It is normal and beneficial to feel sore after weight training. It indicates that your muscles are growing and becoming stronger. The first two weeks seem to be the worst when a previously inactive person begins weight training. Go easy in the beginning so you do not lose the desire to continue.

It is best to consult expert advice on proper stance and positioning. You can check out the services of a certified athletic trainer at your local health club or find a good book with clear pictures, by a well-known authority. Just be aware that an expert on fitness is not always the best advisor on dietary recommendations.

Some weight training sources advise consuming egg whites instead of whole eggs and the use of the artificial sweetener, aspartame. As I stated in **Day 6**, egg yolks have very important ingredients that improve fat metabolism and do not raise cholesterol. Aspartame contains methanol, which is very toxic to the liver and nervous system. Toxic stress to the liver may actually impede weight loss.

Exercise repetition intervals in weight training programs are usually manageable for the average, healthy person. Typical routines involve doing the same exercise with repetitions of twelve, ten, eight, and six with a minute of rest in between each interval. Afterward, one or two more sets of twelve repetitions at a higher intensity are performed on the same muscle group. The entire cycle of repetitions might be too strenuous at first to someone who has been inactive. My advice is to start slowly at whatever capacity you are capable. You will be amazed at your progress in just a month's time.

It is best to concentrate on the upper body one day and the lower body workout on the third day. On the day in between weight training sessions, find an activity that offers a twenty-minute aerobic workout. It is important to take a day of rest every seven days. Therefore, each week should have only three days of weight training, with three days of twenty to forty minutes of aerobic activities in between.

PERSONAL STORY

For two months prior to writing this book, I started following a popular weight-training book to exercise at home with dumbbells, which are inexpensive and very safe to use. I appreciated not having to find time to go to a gym. Many times, over the years, I have joined gyms for short spurts over the winter and lost interest because *nothing changed*. It seemed most gyms ran me through a circuit without allowing enough time on each muscle group.

It has been really exciting to watch the strength in both my body and mind improve. This increase in physical and mental strength has allowed me to move a major obstacle out of my life. For years I have enjoyed writing and teaching about health. It has frustrated me that the health habits I have practiced for twenty-five years still are not public knowledge when so many symptoms and diseases are preventable and reversible!

I knew writing a book was the only way to create the type of "mass action" needed to help people become more effective at caring for their health. Two months after beginning my weight-training program, I took writing my book off my "Can't find the time" list.

What important tasks do you have on your "Can't find the time" list? I not only found time to spend thirty to sixty minutes per day on aerobic activity or weight lifting, but I also found time to write a book. Fulfilling such an important goal has been the most energizing and exciting thing I have done in "umpteen" years.

I challenge you to find time in your day that is presently consumed with non-productive activities that bring you little joy. If nothing else, exercising will relieve some of the guilt of watching TV. For workaholics, taking time to redirect your energy will eventually lead you into a more balanced work life.

TODAY'S ACTIVITY

PREPARATION FOR WEIGHT TRAINING

Choose one of the following activities to get a feel for weight training. Be sure to consult your doctor first to make sure you are capable of this level of exercise:

- Carry a water bottle in each hand when walking. Be sure to drink from each side equally to keep things balanced.
- Put a few grapefruits in a backpack as you go for a walk or hike. Start with a small number and work up to a bigger load. Be sure to measure your pulse and walk at a pace that keeps your heart rate below the level of 180 minus your age as described in Day 12. Even a small amount of weight can create significant changes in your pulse.
- Get two cans of equal weight or some dumbbells. Lie on a bed or floor and hold the cans at your shoulders with your elbows out to your side. Lift the cans slowly, straight upward, until your elbows are straight. Bring the weights back down slowly to the original position. Start out with five or ten repetitions, depending on your comfort level. This exercise is done more efficiently on a bench where your elbows can go a little lower than your chest.
- If you have some strap-on weights, put them on your ankles and try some standing leg lifts to the front, side and back. Hold onto a wall, chair or counter for support. To do a similar exercise without the weights, stand near a corner, facing one wall. Place both hands on the wall and push your foot against the other wall with your leg at about a forty-five-degree angle. Hold it for about five seconds. This is an example of an isometric form of exercise. You can do a similar exercise lifting your leg forty-five degrees behind you (against the wall) by holding onto a chair.
- Grab your cans or dumbbells and do some knee-bends. Keep your back and head straight and only go down to where your thighs are parallel to the floor. If it has been awhile since you have done knee-bends, get used to this exercise first without using weights. You may have to hold onto a chair or counter the first several times.

If you can do these exercises, you are ready for a more organized program. Check your local bookstore, video rental store, or recreation center and find a program that is appropriate for your age, level of fitness and state of health. Even if you started with only one exercise per day, it would still be better than doing nothing. Remember to consult your doctor first if you have any health concerns.

I am convinced that maintaining good health requires us to become stronger and more active. Older teens and adults of all ages benefit from muscle strengthening exercises. It is a form of exercise you do for only minutes per day but receive benefits twenty-four hours per day.

Consider how weight training will alter your sense of power. Becoming stronger physically can do wonders for a person with a low self-esteem or who has been chronically tired or ill. The way you carry yourself gives subconscious messages to both your own mind and those you interact with.

It is difficult to imagine someone like **Arnold Schwarzenegger** moping around feeling lousy. A few years ago, Arnold had heart surgery to repair a congenital defect but it did not seem to have slowed him down. A strong and powerful person like Arnold expects to have a life that is both successful and joyful. All of us can choose to experience life with the same attitude.

"The only questions that really matter
are the ones you ask yourself."
— Ursula L. LeGuin

3 DAY FOOD & ACTIVITY DIARY

	Date:	Date:	Date:
Morning Meal Time:			
Snack			
Noon Meal Time:			
Snack			
Evening Meal Time:			
Snack			
Symptoms (Physical & Emotional)			
Exercise Type & Duration			

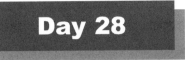

Day 28

"The only place you find success before work is in the dictionary."
— May V. Smith

How's Your Posture?

Many people do not understand the relationship of posture and spinal structure to our health, energy and vitality. We all recognize the effects of aging on posture, such as stooped shoulders and forward posture of the head. These signs can also occur in a much younger person who is depressed, very ill or malnourished. Paying attention to your structure and posture long before your elder years can improve your energy and vitality. It may also help prevent a painful, debilitating posture as you age.

The definition of good posture is when all your muscles are at rest. Therefore, a good posture should not be taxing to any of your muscles. Improving your posture can significantly decrease your fatigue. This can be accomplished with a combination of chiropractic spinal alignment, back strengthening exercises, a good mattress and pillow, and efficient workplace ergonomics.

Occupations where you spend the majority of time standing are the easiest to maintain good posture unless there is frequent lifting or twisting involved. Sitting for long periods often taxes the muscles of the entire spine and head, and a good chair is a must. It should support the curve in the low back, which automatically helps your neck retain its curve. Your computer and work tasks should be at eye level so you are not constantly looking down. Work tasks should allow your arms to feel relaxed.

Your bed pillow is another important consideration for your posture. Many people use too high of a pillow and this, over time, can mold your neck into a forward posture. I recommend pillows that have a foam edge to support the neck curve and allow the base of the head to rest in a soft area lower than the foam edge. These pillows are excellent for both a side-lying and face-up sleep posture. I determine which size foam edge is needed by doing an arm muscle test. Your arm will go weak when the edge is too large. Ask a chiropractor to check which pillow size is best for you.

In order to improve your posture, you cannot just pull your shoulders back. This certainly does not allow the muscles to be at rest. Imagine yourself as a marionette where you have a string pulling up the top of your head. Allow your entire body to be lifted up by this imaginary string. This should change not only how your head is situated but also your breastbone and hips/pelvis. Focus on your breastbone. Is it caved into your chest? As you raise your breastbone, your shoulders will naturally fall more in line with your ear and hip. This should feel less tense. Try to become aware of your posture throughout the day and remember to breathe!

TODAY'S ACTIVITY

CHECK YOUR POSTURE

Buddy up with a friend or family member to do a posture check. Chiropractors look at the posture from both the back and the side. From the side view, your ear, shoulder, hip socket and ankle bone should all be in the same vertical plane. The position of the head is the most common abnormality here.

From the back view, see if one ear lobe appears higher than the other. You may have to lift up their hair to visualize this. Check if you can see more of their jaw or cheek on one side. Compare the height of the two shoulders. Checking the height of the hips often requires you to visualize the waistline to see if one has more of a crease than the other.

Also, notice if the toes turn outward – a common postural fault. This is the result of weakness in a muscle of your low back (the psoas muscle). Sometimes the toes may even turn inward. Notice the inside arch of the feet to determine if they have flattened. Next, have the person bend forward and look to see if one side of the ribcage elevates. This indicates a significant curvature of the thoracic section of the spine, commonly known as scoliosis.

Now, lie horizontally across a bed, face down, and leave your feet hanging off the edge. Ask a family member to check the heels of your shoes with your toes pointing straight downward. See if one leg is shorter than the other one. This usually does not mean your leg is really shorter. Rather, it shows you have numerous distortions in the spine, known as subluxations, which require chiropractic attention to alleviate.

If any imbalances of posture are evident, you should be under the regular care of a chiropractor and begin strengthening your spine with exercises. Chiropractic treatment is not just something to consider when you have spinal pain. It is a system of making the spine more balanced for optimal functioning of the nervous system. Because the nervous system controls the entire body, spinal subluxations can interfere with this function.

This is the major difference between chiropractors and physical therapists. Some physical therapists do a type of manipulation of the spine, but it is usually targeted only toward a specific area of pain or muscle spasm. Most chiropractors treat much more than just the area that hurts. We view the spine as a whole and help make the entire skeletal system, posture and nervous system function more efficiently.

Chiropractic is also great for stress reduction. It is wonderful to see people relax during the treatment and hear feedback later that they are finally sleeping better. Since the majority of illnesses and disease have a stress component, it is great to be able to offer patients a way to tone down that "fight or flight" overdrive that is sometimes difficult to turn off.

Personal Story

I did not see a chiropractor until I was twenty-two years old. I have been receiving chiropractic care at least monthly for twenty-five years now. In that time, I have rarely experienced pain. In fact I have only needed a pain reliever about a dozen times in that entire time period. As I mentioned in the introduction, my complete state of health has improved in that time and I am rarely ill with infections.

Remarkably, the primary reason I changed careers to become a chiropractor was because of a dramatic recovery I received in 1975, while suffering one of my typical sore throats. My throat infections had been very predictable – they always lasted a week. One day, my throat had just started to hurt when a chiropractor came into the dental office where I worked. He suggested my sore throat might heal quicker if I had my spine adjusted. Naturally, having had no experience with this type of health care I thought this suggestion sounded outlandish. But since I did not want to be sick for a week, I decided to give it a try. To my amazement, my sore throat was completely healed by the next morning. I was quite impressed.

He explained that a properly functioning nervous system can help the entire body work better. I certainly noticed an increase in energy and decrease in tension from the chiropractic adjustment. It was a life-changing experience that led me to switch careers. Since that time, I never again needed an antibiotic to chase away infections. Prior to that, I was on a course of antibiotics at least two to three times every year.

I wish I could tell you that in my career I have made everyone's infections go away with a simple adjustment. What I can tell you is that many of my patients with upper respiratory infections have felt better after treatment and used fewer drugs. With the need to avoid overuse of antibiotics, it makes good sense to explore natural, drug-free approaches to minor health problems. Chiropractic treatment, massage, nutrition, acupuncture, herbs, Oriental medicine, etc. all have something of value in treating colds, flu, sinusitis, etc.

Chiropractic is Gentle and Safe

Some people avoid chiropractic care because they fear being hurt by the adjusting techniques that rotate your neck or twist your lower back. Although those methods are very safe, there is one way to put your fears to rest. About thirty years ago, a chiropractic adjusting instrument was developed that adjusts your entire spine without any twisting. It is called the **Activator Method**® of chiropractic.

This technique uses a small, rubber-tipped, spring-loaded instrument to adjust the bones of your spine and extremities. This technique is very safe, effective and painless and should allay the fears of even the most skeptical patient. There are many doctors throughout the world who are certified in this technique. You can find their names and locations on the web site, **www.activator.com,** or by calling **Activator Methods** at (602) 224-0220. I have used this technique my entire career. The superb research done by **Activator Methods** has provided diagnostic criteria that allow doctors an accurate means of correcting subluxations in both the spine and extremities.

Another valuable chiropractic web site is **www.chiroweb.com**. This site is a newspaper distributed to chiropractors throughout the world offering a variety of information on the latest research and health news on chiropractic and natural healing.

TODAY'S ACTIVITY

EXTENSION EXERCISES

Extension is an excellent stretching exercise for strengthening the back muscles that support our posture. The majority of our everyday activities involve flexing or bending at the waist. In order to strengthen any muscle you need to shorten it. Therefore, to strengthen the back you need to extend the spine rather then flexing it.

> Please Note: If you have any pains or weakness in the back please consult your chiropractor or physician first.

This exercise is performed while lying face down on a mat or large towel on the floor. When doing each of the movements, breathe in and then exhale as you come back to your original position. If possible, hold each position for about four seconds before coming back down.

Exercise 1: Lying face down, extend your arms above your head. While breathing in, lift up one arm and your head. Hold four seconds and exhale down. Rest for a second or two before beginning the next movement.

Exercise 2: As you inhale again lift the other arm and your head. Hold four seconds and exhale down.

Exercise 3: Rest a second and then lift up both arms and your head as you inhale. Do not strain. If you are unable to lift either of your arms, ask a friend to gently lift your arm just a couple of inches off the floor. Discontinue these movements if they start to cause any pain.

Exercise 4: Next, you are going to ignore your entire upper body, but remember to breathe! While inhaling, and keeping your knee straight, lift up one leg toward the ceiling. Hold for four seconds and exhale coming down.

Exercise 5: Rest a second and then lift the other leg while inhaling. Hold four seconds and then exhale down.

Exercise 6: Now if you can do this without pain, inhale and lift up both legs for four seconds and exhale down.

Exercise 7: The next step requires concentration because you will be lifting the opposite arm and leg! While inhaling, lift up your left arm and right leg. Hold four seconds and exhale down.

Exercise 8: Inhale again and lift the right arm and the left leg. Hold four seconds and exhale down.

Exercise 9: This last move should only be attempted if your entire back is pain free and not likely to sprain a ligament. Inhale and lift up all four limbs plus your head. Hold for four seconds and exhale down.

EXTENSION EXERCISES

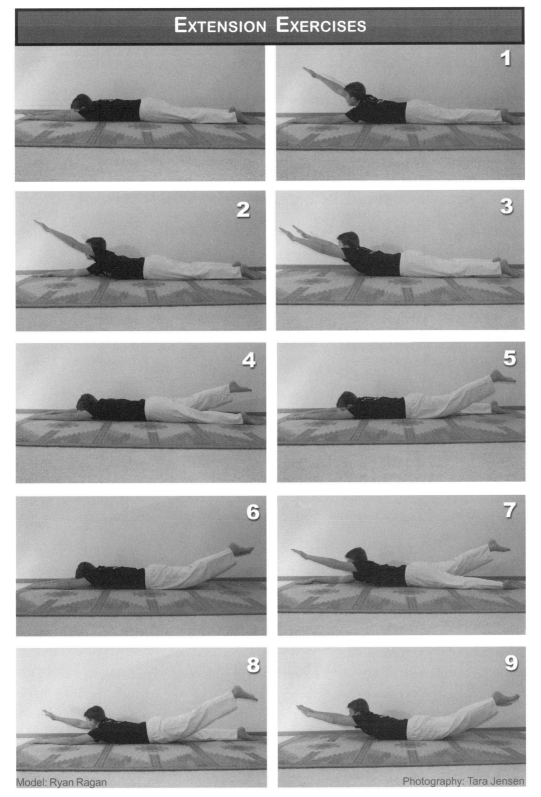

Model: Ryan Ragan

Photography: Tara Jensen

Congratulations! You have completed an entire set of back extension exercises. The first time only do one set to avoid strain. Next time add another set if you feel up to it. Only do what you can handle and avoid stress to muscles or ligaments.

Like the breathing exercises in ***Day 9--Take a Breathing Break***, the extension exercises enhance activity of the parasympathetic nervous system. This is your "rest and digest" nervous system function. Therefore, this would be a great exercise before sitting down to a meal, or for unwinding before bedtime. When your body is in a flexion pose for most of the day, such as sitting or driving, the sympathetic nervous system is very active. This is good, because we do not want to fall asleep while driving! However, sometimes your "fight or flight," high-gear mode does not want to let go. This series of exercises is a great way to calm down.

INFANT POSTURE

Let's digress a bit and talk about infant posture. "What posture?" you ask. They only lie down, roll over and sit up. Ah, but many competitive parents can not wait to see their child walking. They have the mistaken belief that the earlier their child learns to walk relates to how intelligent they are. Bragging about what age their child walked has been popular for at least fifty years! Parents often put babies in various devices such as walkers and jumping harnesses that put them into an upright posture and encourage earlier walking. This is not wise!

Encouraging an upright posture before a child has completed the crawling stage of their neurological development is very stressful to the developing spinal column. It is also confusing and disruptive to the neurologic organization of the brain. It can cause problems in both thinking and motor control, and result in learning disabilities, hyperactivity and clumsiness. Structurally, it can put undue strain on the lower back, before the spine is ready. This may cause postural faults and chronic back pains.

Children must be given ample opportunity to crawl, not being constantly confined to playpens. They should continue crawling until they develop a normal crawling pattern.

My son first crawled in what I refer to as a "GI Joe" pattern. He used his elbows instead of his hands. I just left him to figure it out and eventually he progressed to a normal crawl. I never once encouraged a standing posture and he did not walk until thirteen months of age. However, he is now fifteen and has shown himself to be extremely intelligent and has always demonstrated very integrated and appropriate emotions.

Infants have several stages of neurological development known as "Primitive Neurological Reflexes." Even during breast feeding, a baby is exhibiting one of these reflexes. As soon as the baby's head turns toward the breast, their hands and feet go through various motions that relate to neurological development. Since a breast-fed infant is positioned on both sides equally, this development progresses in a balanced fashion. On the other hand, a parent who is bottle-feeding an infant may always tend to hold the infant with their head to the same side, and this interferes with this stage of neurological development. My advice to bottle-feeding parents is to regularly change the baby's position from one side to the other.

When an adult suffers from a stroke and becomes paralyzed, a physical therapist must lead them through a progression of neurological stages that simulates infant learning. They are first exercised in a crawling pattern before attempting to regain walking function. Recovery is hindered if they do not proceed in this order.

Allowing your child to go through their neurological stages, in the appropriate order, creates balanced development in the brain and nervous system. Allowing "nature to take its course" will help your child become strong and a fast learner. Do not be tempted to buy the various devices that encourage mobility in an upright posture before they have learned to crawl.

HEALTHY BONES FOR GOOD POSTURE

The last thing I want to talk about regarding posture is osteoporosis and the calcium craze. This topic is a subject of much confusion and debate. Vitamin companies would have you believe that you need gigantic quantities of calcium. There are many reasons why Americans suffer from osteoporosis. This disease is much more than inadequate calcium in the diet. Many cultures throughout the world do not consume any dairy. The present generation of American seniors who are suffering from osteoporosis grew up on enormous quantities of dairy products.

Where did we get the idea that bones were only made of calcium? Like anything in nature, several minerals and nutrients work together to make the whole package. Hence, a multivitamin is the first place to start. Taking any mineral by itself will automatically drive every other mineral in the body up or down, creating tremendous imbalance. Whether you need extra calcium in addition to your multivitamin is a decision to made with a doctor who is competent in the subject of nutrition and biochemistry. It should also be based on a bone density exam or a **Bone Resorption Assessment** lab test (available from **Great Smokies Lab**).

Americans should not be self-medicating with calcium via orange juice, antacids or high potency mineral products. Most people are unaware that calcium citrate can be four times more absorbable than calcium gluconate. Therefore, taking 1,500 milligrams of citrate could have the equivalent biochemical action of six thousand milligrams of gluconate. Some health problems, related to excessive calcium in respect to magnesuim, are asthma, constipation, hypertension, kidney stones and cardiovascular plaquing. If you have one of these disorders, you should be wary of taking too much calcium in regard to magnesium. The balance of calcium and magnesium is one of the most important mineral relationships in the body.

Another calcium fad is to promote antacids as a dietary source of calcium. These products contain calcium carbonate, which is basically chalk and is a poorly absorbed form of calcium. The antacid portion of this product produces an alkaline pH, which actually discourages calcium absorption. Calcium is absorbed best with an acid pH. Therefore, taking calcium along with vitamin C or during a meal (where hydrochloric acid is released) enhances its absorption.

The antacid calcium fad came about when the more powerful, acid-blocking drugs were switched in status from prescription-only to over-the-counter. antacid sales were in jeopardy so they changed their focus. One brand of antacid now enjoys greater sales as a calcium supplement than it ever did as an antacid. Marketing is very effective in convincing doctors, dieticians and consumers, but hype does not mean it is valid science.

CALCIUM AND PHOSPHORUS

Another important mineral which exerts a very important effect over your calcium balance is phosphorus. Our bloodstream needs to have a very specific ratio of calcium to phosphorus in order to maintain our acid and alkaline balance. Excess phosphorus causes an increased demand for calcium. This demand often gets met by removing calcium from the bones. High phosphorus content is found in meats, dairy, cereals and soda pop. The wise recommendation for eating meat is to choose a portion similar to a deck of cards.

The phosphoric acid in soda pop is wreaking havoc on the bones of young people. I have seen the osteoporotic "dowager's hump" (round shoulders and bony protrusion at the base of the neck) in people in their thirties who are consuming several sodas per day. Coffee, alcohol, sugar and hydrogenated fats are also major causes of bone depletion. Again, this is why I stress that you cannot afford to ingest any of these risk factors *daily*.

We are making it too tempting for children to destroy their future health by having soda machines prominently located in schools. A survey linking soda consumption and bone fractures was compiled by **Harvard Medical School** and reported in the ***Archives of Pediatric and Adolescent Medicine*** in June 2000. They found that teenage girls who drank carbonated beverages were three times more likely to have a broken bone than those who did not drink them.

Since forty to sixty percent of bone mass is supposed to be *added* during adolescence, it makes no sense to encourage daily consumption of something that robs young bones of their minerals.

> "People are not the best because they work hard.
> They work hard because they are the best."
> — Bette Midler

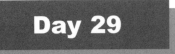

Day 29

"I've learned that the Lord didn't do it all in one day.
What makes me think I can?"

—Andy Rooney

How Are You Sleeping?

Hopefully, as we near the end of this program, the diet and lifestyle changes you have made are providing you with more restful sleep. Getting adequate sleep is one of the most important aspects of your health program. The reason I put this information toward the end of this book is because there are so many factors involved with getting consistent good sleep that need to be taught beforehand.

Before **Thomas Edison** invented the light bulb in 1913, the average American devoted nine hours a night to sleeping. Today, the average is seven and a half hours, with many people getting less. The **National Sleep Foundation** took a survey which found that 64 percent of all Americans get less than eight hours of sleep per day, while thirty-two percent get less than six hours.

It is estimated that insomnia and sleep deprivation are costing American companies $18 billion a year in lost productivity. This survey also found that sixty-one percent of workers said their decision-making suffered after a bad night's sleep, and thirty-seven percent said daytime drowsiness prevented them from doing their best work.

Statistics show that the typical American collects an annual sleep debt of five hundred hours and physically benefits from an afternoon nap. Twenty years ago, a person taking a nap would be fired. Now occupations with safety concerns over high levels of fatigue, such as railroad workers, are considering ten to twenty minute "power naps."

Unfortunately, poor sleep equates to poor health. A Finnish study of more than ten thousand people, over a period of six years, demonstrated that men who had sleeping problems were 250 percent more likely to die during this period than men who slept well. One reason for this decline in health is because the "natural killer" cells of the immune system go into high gear during sleep. This activity drops significantly after only twenty-four hours of sleep deprivation.

Insomnia is the perception of inadequate or poor quality sleep caused by difficulty falling asleep, waking up frequently at night, getting up earlier than desired in the morning or waking up unrefreshed. Insomnia is a major problem among older people and anyone suffering from excessive stress, various diseases or chronic pain. It is also very common during pregnancy, around menstruation and with menopause symptoms such as hot flashes. Sleep disruptions may also be the result of snoring spouses, sleep apnea, light or temperature problems, jet lag and working late or mixed shifts.

TODAY'S ACTIVITY

The following is a short quiz to test your knowledge about sleep. Answer **True** or **False** to the following statements provided by the **National Sleep Foundation**. Check your answers at the end of this chapter.

True False

☐ ☐ 1. During sleep, your brain rests.

☐ ☐ 2. You cannot learn to function normally with one to two fewer hours of sleep a night than you need.

☐ ☐ 3. Boredom makes you feel sleepy, even if you have had enough sleep.

☐ ☐ 4. Resting in bed with your eyes closed cannot satisfy your body's need for sleep.

☐ ☐ 5. Snoring is not harmful as long as it does not disturb others or wake you up.

☐ ☐ 6. Everyone dreams nightly.

☐ ☐ 7. The older you get, the fewer hours of sleep you need.

☐ ☐ 8. Most people do not know when they are sleepy.

☐ ☐ 9. Raising the volume of your radio will help you stay awake while driving.

☐ ☐ 10. Sleep disorders are mainly due to worry or psychological problems.

☐ ☐ 11. The human body never adjusts to night shift work.

☐ ☐ 12. Most sleep disorders go away even without treatment.

PERSONAL STORY

For several years, insomnia was one of the most severe and debilitating symptoms of my autoimmune illness. My sleeplessness was made all the more irritating by one to four hours of hive attacks every night. As if that was not bad enough, in 1986 I awoke one night when a rapist put his hands over my mouth. Luckily, I was able to scream him out of my house before being harmed. My sleep became much worse for the next three years until I moved into an apartment in the same building as my parents. I did not care that I was a grown woman in my thirties. In order to stop feeling afraid I needed the psychological peace of feeling protected by being under the same roof as my parents. I learned to not allow stress or fear interfere with sleep. It is much less stressful to move!

There is absolutely no way you can recover from fatigue or any chronic illness without adequate sleep. You must consider getting adequate sleep as a high priority for your health. Our major growth and repair happens during stage four deep sleep, when we release growth hormone. About two-thirds of men's growth hormone production occurs during deep sleep, while only about one-third of women's does. Do not be misled into thinking you can continue to deprive yourself of sleep and make up for it by taking human growth hormone.

Research by the **University of Chicago**, reported in the ***Journal of the American Medical Association***, in August of 2000, found sleep quality started to deteriorate in men between the ages of twenty-five and forty-five. They found that the proportion of Rapid Eye Movement (REM) sleep dropped from twenty percent of a normal night's sleep for men under twenty-five to less than five percent for those over thirty-five. By age forty-five, few men spend much time in deep sleep. Growth hormone secretion declined by seventy-five percent.

This study suggests the decline in growth hormone starts as much as two decades earlier than previously believed. Decreases in growth hormone production lead to blood sugar imbalances, increased stomach fat, premature aging, loss of muscle mass and decreased exercise capacity.

The study also found that when men reached their fifties, they began releasing more of the stimulatory stress hormone cortisol late at night. High cortisol is believed to mediate the chronic "wear and tear" of the stress response, including memory loss and insulin resistance in aging. Like growth hormone deficiency, cortisol excess is also strongly tied to increased body fat, loss of muscle mass, bone breakdown, and heart disease.

This pattern of increased cortisol at night is also seen in conditions such as chronic fatigue syndrome, fibromyalgia, and other painful conditions. As mentioned in ***Day 19--Low Thyroid and Adrenal Function***, this abnormal pattern can be detected by taking four saliva tests over a twenty-four-hour period in the **Adrenocortex Stress Profile** (available through **Great Smokies Diagnostic Lab** – see Resources).

Although I never had this hormone tested during the worst years of my illness, I suspect my insomnia was very much related to excessive cortisol at night. My insomnia started to improve with a particular adrenal supplement, **Drenatrophin PMG®**, by **Standard Process Labs** (see ***Resources***). I took three to six tablets an hour before bedtime. Most adrenal supplements help you feel more energetic but this is the only adrenal product I have found that helps decrease the "wound too tight" feeling that does not allow your body to fall asleep.

INSOMNIA AND SLEEP DEPRIVATION

Insomnia is an ***involuntary*** loss of sleep. Most people do not realize that they are flirting with disaster by ***voluntarily*** depriving themselves of adequate sleep on a frequent basis. One of the greatest false beliefs of our society is that if we squeeze a few more hours into our waking day we will achieve more. This might be true in the short term but it comes with huge costs over the long term.

Sleep deprivation causes many health problems and disruptions of motor and intellectual functions. After staying awake seventeen to nineteen hours, and still getting five to seven hours of sleep, your performance on simple tasks may be worse than if you were legally drunk, according to research published in the journal, ***Occupational and Environmental Medicine.***

College students have the mistaken belief they are learning more by staying up late, when in reality sleep deprivation causes them to perform poorly on their tests and retain less knowledge. When I was in chiropractic college, I stopped studying every night by 10 PM, despite carrying an average of twenty-five credit hours for eight straight semesters. I always made good grades but the proof of my knowledge retention came when it was time for the National Board exams, for which I studied less than two days, but passed every part of the exams the first time.

THE NEED FOR SLEEP DOES NOT DIMINISH WITH AGE BUT DOES VARY:

- Toddlers need about eleven hours per night, plus a two-hour nap during the day.

- Preschoolers need eleven to twelve hours per night; half of them nap during the day.

- School-age children need about ten hours.

- Teens need an average of 9.5 hours per night. Most get less than 8.5.

- Adults need around eight hours a night. Most get around seven hours on weeknights and 7.5 hours on weekends.

Research shows that when people do not get enough sleep, they build up a "sleep debt." The debt accumulates night after night: Getting one hour less sleep for eight nights in a row will cause your brain to need sleep as desperately as if you had stayed up all night, according to sleep researcher **William Dement** of **Stanford University**, "In the simplest terms, a large sleep debt makes you stupid," says **Dement** in his book, ***The Promise of Sleep***, written with **Christopher Vaughn.**

Drowsiness causes 100,000 car crashes per year, killing thousands of people and injuring many more. It was reported that lack of sleep played a role in such incidents as the Three Mile Island nuclear disaster and the Exxon Valdez oil spill. Forcing medical residents to work excessive numbers of hours has led to medication errors and other serious medical mistakes.

Using medications such as prednisone (cortisone) and some antidepressants can wreak havoc on sleep. Some people use over-the-counter medications such as antihistamines to help sleep but this can cause drowsiness into the next day.

Many prescription sleep medications do not allow your brain to go through the entire four stages of sleep. They put you immediately into stage two sleep and then leave you there. This does not allow your body to get into deep, stage four sleep. This prevents the body from achieving its growth and repair benefits from the release of growth hormone during this time. Ask your doctor and pharmacist about this before deciding to try drug therapy for sleep. The only drug I am aware of that allows you to reach stage four sleep is Ambien (zolpidem). Newer drugs may have been developed that have this benefit.

> ## TIPS TO HELP ENSURE A GOOD NIGHT'S SLEEP:
>
> - Go to bed and get up at the same time every day.
>
> - Be outside without glasses or contacts every morning for at least ten minutes to activate your pineal gland to produce melatonin.
>
> - Exercise regularly but complete the workout at least three hours before bedtime.
>
> - Eat protein at least three hours prior to bedtime.
>
> - Establish a bedtime routine, such as taking a bath, stretching or reading a book. Two cups of Epsom salts or three drops of the essential oil, lavender, in your bath can promote relaxation. Putting a few drops of lavender on your pillow may also be helpful.
>
> - Avoid caffeine *entirely*, not just in the afternoons. This includes coffee, tea, soft drinks and chocolate.
>
> - Avoid nicotine late in the day. Better yet, quit!
>
> - Do not drink alcohol to help you sleep.
>
> - Light exposure during the night disrupts melatonin production and interferes with sleep. Keep the shades drawn and turn off the lights, computer and television.

NATURAL REMEDIES FOR SLEEP

In addition to the adrenal supplement I already mentioned, there are many natural remedies that can help with sleep. Recall the extension exercises described in **Day 28--How's Your Posture?**. Deep breathing exercises and meditation exercises are also extremely valuable to quiet your thoughts and put your mind into more restful brain waves. Listening to a relaxation or meditation tape can allow you to drift off into sleep.

A series of exercises called "**Jacobson Relaxation Technique**" involves lying in bed and first tensing and then relaxing individual sections of the body to release muscle tension. You might start at the feet and squeeze the toes on both feet for a few seconds and then release. Travel to the calves, thighs, buttocks, low back, mid-back, hands, forearms, upper arms, shoulders, neck, mouth, nose, forehead and then scalp. If necessary, repeat the entire process.

According to Oriental Medicine, when people suffer a particular symptom at the same time nearly every day, you can trace the problem to a particular acupuncture meridian or organ function. Patients have often told me they awaken with insomnia around the same time every night. In the time period of 11 PM to 1 AM, we can trace that to the gall bladder meridian. The liver meridian is most active from 1 AM to 3 AM. This is one of the more frequent times people awaken due to the liver being overburdened with its nightly detoxification duties.

Waking during a particular time period can also relate to an emotional conflict associated with the meridian. I recently had a patient who kept waking up at 4 AM. This was the time (3 – 5 AM) when the lung meridian is most active. This meridian has to do with grief which was an issue she was presently focusing on because of a recent near-death of an elderly loved one. She started sleeping better when the acupuncture point associated with this function was treated. Also, waking during the liver's peak time may be related to an anger issue.

Various vitamins, minerals and herbs can help sleep disturbances. **Standard Process Labs (SPL)** is one of the only nutrient companies that separates their B vitamins into those that are alcohol-soluble (**Cataplex® B**) and those that are alcohol-insoluble (**Cataplex® G**). This is helpful for treating very specific symptoms related to B vitamin deficiencies where using the whole B complex would not be as effective. I have found that problems with nocturnal urination and waking with difficulty falling back asleep are often helped by **Cataplex® B**. **Cataplex® G** is often useful when you have leg jerks prior to falling asleep or the sensation of hearing your heartbeat on your pillow.

Nightmares are a sign of needing better elimination of ammonia (from protein metabolism) and can often be helped by **SPL's A-C Carbamide®.** When you cannot recall your dreams, this may be a sign of B6 deficiency. Excessive dreaming with too much action can be a sign of manganese deficiency. Be careful with manganese supplementation. Do not take extra for more than a couple of months due to toxicity issues.

Herbs that are helpful for sleep and relaxation include valerian root, passion flower, hops and kava kava root. Sleep can also be helped by both calcium and magnesium. **Metagenics** makes a product with each of these ingredients called **MyoCalm P.M.™**. If muscle spasm or anxiety are the biggest problems keeping you from relaxing, kava kava may be the best choice. **Metagenics** has an excellent product called **Kava Plus™**. One of the ways you can tell if a kava supplement is of good quality is if tasting the tablet causes a sharp biting sensation on your tongue.

Melatonin is not something I often recommend as a supplement, especially for people younger than age forty or those with immune diseases. I prefer that people try to increase their melatonin naturally, such as with early morning walks. It may be useful for short-term situations such as jet-lag or for someone who does shift work and has difficulty getting enough sleep.

> "Dream big and dare to fail."
> — Norman D. Vaughan

QUIZ ANSWERS

1. **False.** While your body rests, your brain does not. An active brain during sleep prepares you for alertness and peak functioning the next day.

2. **True.** The need for sleep is biological. While children need more sleep than adults, how much sleep any individual needs is genetically determined. Most adults need eight hours of sleep to function at their best. How do you determine what you need? On a night you feel fairly well rested, try sleeping until you wake up on your own. Feel rested? The length of time you slept is your sleep need.

3. **False.** Boredom does not cause sleepiness; it merely unmasks sleep loss.

4. **True.** Sleep is as necessary to health as food and water, and rest is no substitute for sleep. Sleep is an active process needed for health and alertness. When you do not get the sleep you need, your body builds up a sleep debt, which eventually must be paid.

5. **False.** Snoring may indicate the presence of a life-threatening sleep disorder called sleep apnea, where you snore loudly and awaken repeatedly during the night, gasping for breath. There is effective treatment--consult a physician.

6. **True.** Dreaming occurs for every person, every night.

7. **False.** Older people may wake up more frequently through the night or sleep less, but they need no less sleep than during young adulthood. Sleep difficulties are not a normal part of aging, but are all too common.

8. **True.** Many people do not know whether they are sleepy, when they are sleepy or why they are sleepy. When driving, do not think you can tough it out if you are sleepy, but only a few miles from your destination. If you are sleepy enough, you can fall asleep anywhere.

9. **False.** Research shows that loud radios, chewing gum and open windows fail to keep sleepy drivers alert. The only short-term solution is to pull over at a safe place and take a short nap or have a caffeine drink.

10. **False.** Stress is the number one reason people report occasional insomnia, but chronic sleep disorders have a variety of causes.

QUIZ ANSWERS CONTINUED

11. **True.** All living things have a circadian, or twenty-four-hour cycle. This affects when we feel sleepy and when we feel alert. Light-and-dark cycles set these circadian rhythms. For a shift worker, the light-and-dark cycle does not change, so the circadian rhythm never adjusts. Whether you work the night shift or not, you are most likely to feel sleepy between midnight and 6 AM And no matter how many years you work a night shift, sleeping during the day remains difficult. Shift workers should avoid caffeine during the last half of the day, block out noise and light at bedtime, and stay away from alcohol and alerting activities before bed.

    Dr. Walker's note: Anyone with a chronic illness should stop working the night shift. Your body needs to get back to a normal, natural circadian rhythm to recover.

12. **False.** Sleep disorders do not disappear without treatment. Untreated sleep disorders can have serious effects such as: worsening of quality of life, school and work performance, and relationships. Untreated sleep disorders can lead to accidents and death.

"Always use the word impossible
with the greatest caution."
--Werner Von Braun

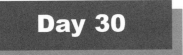

Day 30

"He who conquers himself has won a greater victory than he who conquers a city."

— Proverbs

"Graduation Day"--Reevaluation

Congratulations! You have made it through thirty days of learning tremendous skills to enhance your health, energy, and vitality. By reading this entire book you now know more about nutrition and natural healing than many of the health practitioners in this country!

With this information you can appreciate that diet, inactivity and stress are the biggest obstacles to conquer. None of these three factors can be changed by anyone but you. This book is a roadmap for a lifelong journey where you will constantly be adapting and learning new tools to improve your health.

You are in charge of your well-being and your future. No one can make you healthy if you are not practicing good health habits. Vibrant energy is not achieved passively or from wishful thinking. It is the result of taking action and making better choices.

My greatest desire is for this book to have given you hope. I want you to realize you can be more in command of your present and future health by employing new information and lifestyle skills. By understanding how to positively impact your health you can achieve a greater level of control over all sickness and disease. You can prevent fatigue from turning into a serious illness that is much more difficult to overcome.

With knowledge comes power. You now have the power to be an active partner with your doctors and other healthcare practitioners. Healing therapies in combination with your efforts will create a synergy that will produce **much greater results than either one alone!** Hopefully, you can achieve greater wellness, vitality and longevity with fewer drugs and surgeries.

Do you recall one of my goals was to help you feel like less of a victim? Victims feel weak and think their only hope is to be rescued. You now have the tools to rescue yourself. You can be more energetic and productive and help your family members and loved ones achieve similar benefits. You no longer have to just let your life happen, you can make it happen.

Today is your graduation day--now is the time to reevaluate how far you have come. Fill out the toxicity quiz completely before looking back at your previous score in **Day 1--Are You Tired or Toxic?** No peeking!

TOXICITY QUESTIONNAIRE
©1997 HealthComm International, Inc. and Immuno Laboratories, Inc. Permission to reprint R9/12/97

Rate the following symptoms based upon your health profile for the past week.

Point scale

0 – **Never** or **almost never** have the symptom
1 - **Occasionally** have it, effect is **not severe**
2 - **Occasionally** have it, effect is **severe**
3 - **Frequently** have it, effect is **not severe**
4 - **Frequently** have it, effect is **severe**

HEAD
_____ Headaches
_____ Faintness
_____ Dizziness
_____ Insomnia   Total _____

EYES
_____ Watery or itchy eyes
_____ Swollen, reddened, or sticky eyelids
_____ Bags or dark circles under eyes
_____ Blurred or tunnel vision (does not include near– or far-sightedness)
                                                                        Total _____

EARS
_____ Itchy ears
_____ Earaches, ear infections
_____ Drainage from ear
_____ Ringing in ears, hearing loss   Total _____

NOSE
_____ Stuffy nose
_____ Sinus problems
_____ Hay fever
_____ Sneezing attacks
_____ Excessive mucus formation   Total _____

MOUTH /THROAT
_____ Chronic coughing
_____ Gagging, frequent need to clear throat
_____ Sore throat, hoarseness, loss of voice
_____ Swollen or discolored tongue, gums, lips
_____ Canker sores   Total _____

SKIN
_____ Acne
_____ Hives, rashes, dry skin
_____ Hair loss
_____ Flushing, hot flashes
_____ Excessive sweating   Total _____

HEART
_____ Irregular or skipped heartbeat
_____ Rapid or pounding heartbeat
_____ Chest pain   Total _____

LUNGS
- —— Chest congestion
- —— Asthma, bronchitis
- —— Shortness of breath
- —— Difficulty breathing   Total _____

DIGESTIVE TRACT
- —— Nausea, vomiting
- —— Diarrhea
- —— Constipation
- —— Bloated feeling
- —— Belching, passing gas
- —— Heartburn
- —— Intestinal/stomach pain   Total _____

JOINTS/ MUSCLE
- —— Pain or aches in joints
- —— Arthritis
- —— Stiffness or limitation of movement
- —— Pain or aches in muscles
- —— Feeling of weakness or tiredness   Total _____

WEIGHT
- —— Binge eating/drinking
- —— Craving certain foods
- —— Excessive weight
- —— Compulsive eating
- —— Water retention
- —— Underweight   Total _____

ENERGY/ ACTIVITY
- —— Fatigue, sluggishness
- —— Apathy, lethargy
- —— Hyperactivity
- —— Restlessness   Total _____

MIND
- —— Poor memory
- —— Confusion, poor comprehension
- —— Poor concentration
- —— Poor physical coordination
- —— Difficulty in making decisions
- —— Stuttering or stammering
- —— Slurred speech
- —— Learning disabilities   Total _____

EMOTIONS
- —— Mood swings
- —— Anxiety, fear, nervousness
- —— Anger, irritability, aggressiveness
- —— Depression   Total _____

OTHER
- —— Frequent illness
- —— Frequent or urgent urination
- —— Genital itch or discharge   Total _____

GRAND TOTAL _____

	Before	After
Day 1: Now go back and check your initial Toxicity Quiz score:	_____	_____
Also, check over your health goals and see if you want to make some changes. Did you meet your one-month goals?	Yes	No
Do your one-year goals seem more attainable than they may have thirty days ago?	Yes	No
Day 2: Have you been consistently taking the "Big 3"?	Yes	No
If yes, have they impacted your energy and vitality?	Yes	No
Day 3: Have you been faithfully writing down your foods, etc.?	Yes	No
Has this helped you improve your eating habits?	Yes	No
Have you been consistent with daily activity?	Yes	No
Day 4: Are you consuming fresher and less processed foods?	Yes	No
Day 5: Has a reduction of sugar improved your energy level?	Yes	No
Have you inspired your family or friends to eat less sugar?	Yes	No
Day 6: Have you felt more energy from getting adequate protein?	Yes	No

Day 8: Go back and reexamine your list of unhealthy habits. See how well you met each of your goals and take the time to set some new ones.

- Recall the person you chose to forgive and see if thinking about that person now brings up the same feelings as when you first wrote their name. Perhaps, you can choose another person to forgive.

- Consider if you have broken any patterns of dishonesty. Notice the sense of relief you feel from no longer conducting your life under that stress.

- If self-hatred was an issue for you, consider how you now feel towards yourself. Look in the mirror and say about yourself, "I love and accept myself just the way I am." Notice whether it feels different than how you felt before.

- Consider whether you have become more loving or tolerant of others, especially those you previously ignored.

	Before	After
Day 9: Have you been taking time for deep breathing?	Yes	No
Day 10: Have you been consuming green foods more often?	Yes	No
Day 11: Have your bowel habits become more normal?	Yes	No
Day 12: Have you been increasing your activity every week?	Yes	No
Have you been trying new activities for variety?	Yes	No
Day 13: Do you have fewer dysbyosis symptoms?	Yes	No

Day 14: Are you consuming little or no refined flours?	Yes	No
Are you noticing your waistline getting slimmer?	Yes	No
Day 15: Have you decreased or eliminated dairy from your diet?	Yes	No
Are your sinuses, lungs or abdomen feeling better?	Yes	No
Day 16: Are you consuming enough water?	Yes	No
Have you eliminated any symptoms of dehydration?	Yes	No
Day 17: Are you getting your four to six servings of vegetables daily?	Yes	No
Day 18: Have you given up the daily use of stimulants?	Yes	No
Do you use stimulants rarely or not at all?	Yes	No
Day 19: Are you getting enough iodine to nourish your thyroid?	Yes	No
Have you decreased drinking ice-cold beverages?	Yes	No
Are you avoiding activities that stress your adrenals?	Yes	No
Day 20: Are you managing your stress better?	Yes	No
Day 21: Are you meditating at least five minutes daily?	Yes	No
Day 22: Are you more aware of expansive and contractive foods?	Yes	No
Has it helped your mental and emotional health?	Yes	No
Day 23: Have you made an effort to avoid hydrogenated fats?	Yes	No
Day 24: Is your digestion improving?	Yes	No
Day 25: Have you become less angry and irritable?	Yes	No
Day 26: Have you eliminated any detoxification symptoms?	Yes	No
Day 27: Are you making plans to start weight training?	Yes	No
Day 28: Have you tried the extension exercises?	Yes	No
Day 29: Have you identified any obstacles to sleeping well?	Yes	No
Day 30: Do you have more desire to take better care of yourself?	Yes	No
Have you had more energy for your loved ones?	Yes	No

If the majority of your check marks are Yes, you are well on your way to making the changes necessary to live your life with energy, vitality and good health. The No answers are the places where you still need to direct your attention. Perhaps now is the time to start the entire program again, so you can learn it from a new perspective.

As I had promised, achieving high energy and good health is not attained by one "magic bullet." Only by making many, small changes in multiple areas of your life, will you achieve your highest level of improvement. Remember, health is a choice. The more obstacles to good health you choose to overcome, the better you will feel.

CONCLUSION

I finished this book the weekend before Thanksgiving. This American holiday is my favorite celebration of the year because it is inclusive of every faith and creed. Everyone celebrates Thanksgiving and there is no concern "political correctness."

Thanksgiving is particularly inspiring because it invites us to consider the people, events and circumstances we have to be thankful for. Counting our blessings can help us appreciate the many little things that bring joy and meaning into our lives. You can also be thankful for what you do not have. Look around in your immediate vicinity or in other countries of the world and be grateful you do not have their struggles.

I am very thankful to have had the opportunity to share my knowledge and experience with you in this book. Although no one enjoys being sick or tired, in some cases our greatest blessings come from overcoming large obstacles. I have met many cancer survivors who were very grateful for the lessons they received from the abrupt wakeup call a serious health challenge offers.

It is my greatest privilege to give God the glory for the many blessings in my life. This was not always the case. I used to put more energy into blaming Him for my problems. I was so angry toward God in the initial years of my illness. I wondered how He could allow me to suffer so much.

For a long time, I wrestled with my emotions. Unlike Job, from the Bible, I was not a very patient and faithful person. Eventually, my negative thoughts led to feelings of hatred and retaliation. What better way to get back at God than to throw my life away? I contemplated suicide.

Perhaps many of you reading this book can relate to a time when you also felt this desperate about your health problems. It is my sincere desire that this information has given you the hope and faith that your health is capable of improving.

The turning point between life and death for me had "God's Plan" written all over it. Giving birth to a healthy son was a momentous event that affirmed to me that my body could still do some things right. My precious child brought joy to the dark days and gave me a greater desire to be victorious.

Having a child at the lowest time in my life taught me to surrender and ask God for His grace and blessings. It helped me relinquish my pride and belief that I was the only one I could depend on. Best of all, it allowed me to experience unconditional love in a way that is the closest thing to God's love for each of us.

Sixteen years later, I can say my life progressed according to His plan. My child has always been a source of tremendous joy and blessings and never felt like a burden. Since his conception, I have no longer had thoughts that life, despite its challenges, was not worth living. My healing has progressed to the point where I now have many gifts to share with the "sick and tired" of the world.

I hope this book has taught you to honor the body you were so richly blessed with. Choose foods as if you were feeding God, Himself. Build your strength with exercise as if you were in basic training for an important mission. When you have the energy and vitality that your body was designed for, you will be able to bless others with unique gifts only you can deliver.

Your greatest treasure is your health. Abundant energy allows you to live every day to the fullest. How you nuture your health today has everything to do with how you will feel ten to fifty years from now. If the information in this book helps you to work productively and enjoy recreation well into your eighties and nineties, I will have certainly succeeded. Enjoy life, and bring joy to others. Let your light shine. Cherish your health.

> "Therefore, as God's chosen people, holy and dearly loved,
> clothe yourselves with compassion, kindness, humility, gentleness and patience.
> Bear with each other and forgive whatever grievances
> you may have against one another. Forgive as the Lord forgave you.
> And over all these virtues put on love,
> which binds them all together in perfect unity."
> — Colossians 3:12-14

Resources

For more information or to purchase the health products recommended in this book, please contact the health professional who referred this book to you.

- For health consultations with Dr. Walker, to purchase books and **Metagenics** products, or to find out more about our clinic services, call toll free (888) 764-2151, locally (970) 224-0774 or visit our web site at **www.vitalitydoctor.com**. That site can also be reached from a link at **www.conquerfatigue.com**.

- To be put on our mailing list, or receive information, please contact us by telephone, email **vitalitydoctor@aol.com**, or by writing:
  Vitality Doctor, 1700 South College, Suite C, Fort Collins, CO 80525

- We welcome your comments on this book. Please write to the Vitality Doctor address above or **conquerfatigue@aol.com**.

Please note: Some of the medical foods for detoxification mentioned in this book are not listed on our web site because Dr. Walker feels that they should be used under the supervision of a licensed health care professional.

COMPANIES OR WEB SITES LISTED IN THIS BOOK

Activator® Methods Chiropractic
PO Box 80317
Phoenix, AZ 85060
(602) 224-0220
general@activator.com
www.activator.com

Alternatives™ For The Health Conscious Individual
Dr. David Williams
Phillips Publishing
7811 Montrose Rd
Potomac, MD 20854
(800) 527-3044
www.DrDavidWilliams.com

The Broda Barnes Foundation
PO Box 110098
31 Prospect Ave.
Trumbull, CT 06611
(203) 261-2101
info@BrodaBarnes.com
www.BrodaBarnes.org

Cell Tech Inc.
Distributors for Super Blue Green® Algae
1300 Main Street
Klamath Falls, OR 97601
(800) 800-1300
feedback@celltech.com
www.celltech.com
To order at a discount as a preferred customer or to become a distributor, please use Dr. Walker's number: 150798

Center for Science in the Public Interest
Nutrition Action Healthletter
1875 Connecticut Avenue, N.W., Suite 300
Washington, D.C. 20009-5728
(202) 332-9110
cspi@cspinet.org
www.cspinet.org

Crook, Dr. William, Author
Professional Books
P.O. Box 3246
Jackson, TN 38303
(901) 660-5027
DrCrookIHF@aol.com
www.candida-yeast.com

Great Smokies Diagnostic Lab (GDSL)
63 Zillicoa St.
Asheville, NC 28801-1074
(800) 522-4762
www.gdsl.com

Healthy Answers Magazine
Advanced Nutrician Publications
11498 Pierce St., Suite A
Riverside, CA 92505
(888) 690-8500
(909) 351-7872

International Association for Colon Hydrotherapy (I-ACT)
P.O. Box 461285
San Antonio, TX 78246-1295
(210) 366-2888
Healthy Answers Magazine
Advanced Nutrition Publications
11498 Pierce St., Suite A
Riverside, CA 92505
(888) 690-8500
(909) 351-7872

Institute for Functional Medicine
PO Box 1729
Gig Harbor, WA 98335
(800) 228-0622
(253) 858-4724
www.fxmed.com

IPS/Health Coach ®
100 Avenida La Pata
San Clemente, CA 92673
(800) 348-1549
(909) 351-7869

Learning Strategies Corporation
900 East Wayzata Blvd
(800) 735-8273
(952) 476-9200
Info@learningstrategies.com
www.learningstrategies.com

Macrobiotics America
David and Cindy Briscoe
720 Bird Street
Oroville, CA 95965
(877) 622-2637
(530) 532-0824
www.macroamerica.com

Metagenics®, Inc.
100 Avenida La Pata
San Clemente, CA 92673
(800) 692-9400
(949) 366-0818
www.metagenics.com

National Sleep Foundation
1522 K Street, Suite 500, NW
Washington D.C. 20005
(202) 347-3472
www.sleepfoundation.org/default.html

Springreen Products, Inc.
PO Box 34710
North Kansas City, MO 64116
(800) 544-8147
(816) 221-3719

Standard Process Labs
1200 West Royal Lee Drive
PO Box 904
Palmyra, WI 531-0904
(800) 848-5061
(262) 495-2122
info@standardprocess.com
www.standardprocess.com

Super Blue Green® Algae
See Cell Tech Inc. above

Permissions

We wish to thank the following sources for permission to use the items listed:

Introduction:

- Cathy cartoon, Courtesy of Universal Press Syndicate, 4520 Main Street, Kansas City, MO, 64111

Day 1:

- Statistics on environmental poisons – Courtesy of Metagenics, Inc. 100 Avenida La Pata, San Clemente, CA 92673, (800) 692-9400
- Toxicity Questionnaire – Courtesy of Health Comm International, Inc., PO Box 1729, Gig Harbor, WA 98335 and Immuno Laboratories
- Cathy cartoon – Courtesy of Universal Press Syndicate (listed above)

Day 2:

- Nutrient-Depleting Substances and The Multivitamin/mineral quiz, Courtesy of *Healthy Answers*, Winter 2000, Advanced Nutrition Publications Inc., 11498 Pierce St., Suite A, Riverside, CA 92505 (888) 690-8500

Day 4:

- The Major Food Additives to Avoid – Courtesy of Center for Science in The Public Interest, Nutrition Action Healthletter, 1875 Connecticut Avenue, N.W., Suite 300, Washington, D.C. 20009-5728

Day 5:

- Sugar Where You Least Expect It – Courtesy of *Lick The Sugar Habit* by Dr. Nancy Appleton, PO Box 3083, Santa Monica, CA 90403
- The Insulin-Glucagon Axis, Determining Your Sensitivity to Insulinogenic Foods, and Carbohydrate Classifications of Fruits and Vegetables – Courtesy of *Choosing Health, The Food Equivalent System*, ©1996, Dr. Mark Percival, IPS/Health Coach®, 100 Avenida La Pata, San Clemente, CA 92673
- Cathy cartoon – Courtesy of Universal Press Syndicate (listed above)

Day 6:

- Quality Proteins – Courtesy of *Choosing Health, The Food Equivalent System*, ©1996, Dr. Mark Percival
- Biologic Values of Dietary Proteins and information on whey protein concentrate – "The Diverse Role of High Quality Protein in Human Health," by David O. Lucas, Ph.D, *Clinical Nutrition Insights*, ©1999, Courtesy of Advanced Nutrition Publications, Inc., 11498 Pierce St., Suite A, Riverside, CA 92505 (888) 690-8500

Day 7:

- Information for this chapter - Courtesy of the *Elemental Analysis Hair Interpretive Guidelines* by Great Smokies Diagnostic Laboratory, 63 Zillicoa Street, Asheville, N.C., 28801

Day 9:

- Evy McDonald's story, from the song "Unconditional Love (The Story of Evy)," from the CD "The Shootout at the I'm OK, You're OK Corral," ©1992 – Courtesy of Greg Tamblyn, Tunetown Records, PO Box 45258, Kansas City, Missouri 64171.
- Amy Graham's story - Courtesy of Chicken Soup For The Soul, Mark Victor Hansen and Jack Canfield

Day 11:

- Pulse Rate as a Predictor of Cardiovascular Deaths – Courtesy of *Alternatives™ For The Health Conscious Individual*, May, 1999, by Dr. David Williams, Phillips Publishing.

Day 12:

- Functions of beneficial bacteria flora, Properties of the NCFM™ Strain of *Lactobacillus acidophilus*, Properties of *Bifidobacteria* – Courtesy of Metagenics, Inc.

Day 13:

- The Dysbiosis Questionnaire, adapted from W.G. Crook, *Tired-So Tired! and the Yeast Connection*, Courtesy of Professional Books, ©2001, Jackson, TN.
- Printout of Case 1 CDSA - Courtesy of Great Smokies Diagnostic Lab (listed above)

Day 14:

- Lactose Intolerance in Ethnic Populations, Common Sources of Lactose, and Nondairy High-Calcium Foods - Courtesy of *Clinical Nutrition: A Functional Approach*, © 1999, Dr. Jeffrey Bland, The Institute For Functional Medicine™, Inc.

Day 16:

- Types of Illnesses Related to Pools and Spas – Courtesy of Colorado State University Environmental Quality Laboratory

Day 17:

- Phytonutrient Color Chart – Courtesy of Dr. Paul Price II, Arvada, Colorado
- ORAC Values and Benefits for Fruits and Vegetables and pesticide residues, reprinted from *Alternatives™ For The Health Conscious Individual*, April, 1999, by Dr. David Williams and its original source – Agriculture Research, February, 1999.
- Cathy cartoon – Courtesy of Universal Press Syndicate (listed above)

Day 19:

- The Basal Temperature Chart - Courtesy of the Broda Barnes Foundation, (203) 261-2101

Day 20:

- Characteristics of Resiliency – Courtesy of *The Survivor Personality*, by Al Siebert, Ph.D, Perigree Books/Berkeley Publishing Group 1996

Day 23:

- Information on trans fats – From *Compiled Notes on Clinical Nutrition Products*, 2nd Edition, Chapters 16 and 17, Courtesy of Walter H. Schmitt, Jr., D.C., AKSP, 1926 Overland Drive, Chapel Hill, N.C. 27514

Day 24:

- The 4 R™ Program – Courtesy of Dr. Jeffrey Bland, The Institute for Functional Medicine, PO Box 1729, Gig Harbor, WA 98335, (800) 228-0662
- Digestive Questions – Courtesy of Metagenics, Inc. 100 Avenida La Pata, San Clemente, CA 92673, (800) 692-9400

Day 25:

- Liver Detoxification, from Detoxification: A Naturopathic Perspective, Joseph E. Pizzorno, N.D. and Michael T. Murray, N.D., Natural Medicine Journal, May 1998, Courtesy of Dr. Michael Murray, www.doctormurray.com

Day 26:

- Information on colon irrigation – Courtesy of the International Association for Colon Hydrotherapy, PO Box 461285, San Antonio, TX 78246-1295, (210) 366-2888
- Cathy cartoon – Courtesy of Universal Press Syndicate (listed above)

Day 29:

- The Sleep Quiz – Courtesy of the National Sleep Foundation, 1522 K Street, Suite 500, NW, Washington, D.C. 20005 (202) 347-3471

Day 30:

- Toxicity Questionnaire – Courtesy of Health Comm International, Inc., PO Box 1729, Gig Harbor, WA 98335 and Immuno Laboratories

Index

aspartame 30, 171, 197

aspirin 11, 184

Association for Applied Psychophysiology and Biofeedback 156

asthma 4, 10, 22, 75, 94, 114, 145, 163, 169, 207

astragalus 78, 80, 148

athlete's foot 99, 107, 125

Attention Deficit Disorder vi, 19, 24, 29, 54, 57, 138, 159

Attention Deficit/Hyperactivity Disorder 26, 29, 159

autoimmune diseases 9, 65, 169, 173

B

backaches 98

bacteria 15, 50, 81, 82, 84, 86, 87, 97, 101, 107, 124, 125, 174

Baker, Dr. Sidney, M.D. 60

barley malt 34, 46

Barnes, Dr. Broda, M.D. 142

Basal Body Temperature Test, The 142

belching 4, 100, 175

Benson, Dr. Herbert 155

bentonite 88, 191

benzpyrene 183

berberine 104

beta blockers 143

beta carotene 16, 21, 22, 24, 176

beta-glucuronidase 85

betaine 30, 184, 185

BHA 30

BHT 30

bifidobacteria 85, 86, 176
    bifidobacterium infantis 85
    bifidus 85, 123, 171, 176
    bifidus infantis 86, 176

bile 2, 81, 86, 87, 176, 181

bilirubin 180

biochemical imbalance 42, 159

biofeedback 93, 156

Biological Value (BV) 48, 50

BioPureProtein 50

biotin 11, 17, 21, 22, 41, 84

birth control pills 11, 99, 115, 181

birth defects 18, 19, 20
    birth deformities 30, 76
    low birth weight 19, 22, 72, 151
    premature 19, 22, 25

bladder 2, 64, 112, 120, 130, 182

Bland, Dr. Jeffrey, Ph.D. iv, 45, 78, 115, 117, 173, 176, 177, 185, 228

bloating 83, 97, 100, 113, 114, 175

blood 2, 9, 22, 25, 26, 75, 119, 142, 180, 181

blood pressure 10, 30, 37, 69, 93, 133, 134, 144, 146, 147, 148, 149, 163, 177

blood sugar 24, 36, 38, 42, 43, 45, 46, 50, 51, 80, 109, 112, 127, 133, 145, 146, 147, 211

blue green algae 162, 164

body fat 49, 195, 196, 211

Bone Resorption Assessment 207

bones 80, 115, 119, 143, 165, 195, 207, 208, 211

bottle-fed 113

bowel 22, 83, 84, 85, 87, 102, 109, 120, 149, 175, 188, 191

brain 10, 13, 24, 25, 30, 36, 41, 42, 53, 76, 97, 119, 131, 137, 138, 150, 156, 164, 182, 207, 210, 212, 213

Brassica family 183, 184

breast cancer 22, 50, 120

breast feeding 49, 206
    breast-fed 25, 113

breathing 2, 4, 27, 69, 93, 119, 120, 188, 206, 220

Brecher, Arline 36

Briscoe, David 77, 159

British Medical Journal 71

Broda Barnes Foundation 144, 225, 228

bromelain 187

bronchitis 64

butyrate 86

BV. See Biological Value

C

C Reactive Protein 37

cadmium 53, 56

caffeine 2, 9, 11, 30, 32, 61, 120, 133, 134, 138, 145, 146, 148, 153, 163, 171, 175, 181, 182, 183, 187

calcium 10, 11, 17, 18, 19, 21, 50, 57, 58, 113, 116, 134, 170, 207, 208

cancer vii, ix, 1, 9, 12, 16, 20, 22, 23, 30, 31, 38, 50, 71, 76, 84, 85, 8797, 108, 109, 120, 123, 125, 127, 130, 149, 169, 171, 179, 181, 182, 183, 185, 186, 189, 190, 192, 193, 222

Cancer Prevention Diet, The 165

Candida 97, 98, 105, 107

Canfield, Jack 67, 229

capillary strength 132

caprylic acid 104, 106

carbohydrates 22, 33, 37, 40, 43, 75, 113, 145, 161

carbon dioxide 75, 86

carcinogenic 30

carcinogens 183, 184, 189

cardiovascular 16, 24, 35, 54, 93, 169, 207

carotenes 128

carotenoids 16, 24, 31, 128, 130

casein 49, 113, 114, 115

castor oil 188

Cataplex B 214

Cataplex G 214

CCR. See Consumer Confidence Report

CDSA. See Comprehensive Digestive Stool Analysis

Cedars-Sinai Medical Center 151

Cell Tech, Inc. 79, 164, 225

cellulases 176

Center for Science in the Public Interest. See CSPI

Centers for Disease Control 35, 72

Institute for Functional Medicine, Inc. iv, 45, 78, 173, 177, 226

insulin 24, 25, 36, 37, 46, 59, 112, 133, 145, 171, 196

insulin resistance 35, 37, 38, 42, 45, 170, 171, 211

International Agency for Research of Cancer 30

International Association for Colon Hydrotherapy 193, 226, 228

intestine 2, 4, 13, 17, 86, 102, 107, 108, 170

intestinal permeability 173, 174, 177

intestine, Large. See colon

intestine, small 64, 112, 189, 190

intrinsic factor 176

inulin 176

iodine 18, 21, 22, 57, 77, 141, 171, 221

iron 11, 12, 17, 18, 19, 21, 41, 134, 146

Irons, V.E. 191, 192

irritability 75, 98, 100, 143, 221

irritable bowel syndrome 107, 143, 174

isoflavones 50, 51, 128

itching ii, 100, 104, 125

Itraconazole 104

J

Jacobsen Relaxation Technique 213

Johns Hopkins 97, 136, 164

joint 25, 169

joints 119, 187

Journal of American Medicine 83

Journal of Gerontology 195

Journal of Obstetrics and Gynocology 15, 86

Journal of the American Dietetic Association 120

Journal of the American Medical Association 12, 53, 211

K

Katke, Michael 175

kava kava 214

Kava Plus 214

Kellogg, Dr. 83

kidney 2, 3, 13, 64, 112, 120, 134, 144, 182

dialysis 85

failure 93

stones 207

Klebsiella 105, 106, 191

Kreb's Cycle 41, 42

Kushi, Michio 165

L

l-carnitine 24, 93

L-glutamine 176, 177

lactate 86

lactic acid 85

lactobacillus 15, 85, 176

lactose 17, 34, 44, 45, 85, 113, 114, 115

intolerance 86, 113, 114

LaLanne, Jack iv, 195

Larson, Dr. Joan Mathews, Ph.D. 29, 59, 60

Lauer, Dr. Michael 94

laxatives 171

LDH 180

lead 53, 56, 122, 124

leaky gut syndrome 171, 173

learning disabilities 5, 30, 206

lethargic 120

leukemia 67

Lick the Sugar Habit 30, 34, 227

licorice root 148, 177

LicoricePlus 148

lifestyle 145, 189, 209

limonene 128, 184, 185

lipases 176

Lipo-Gen 87, 185

lipoic acid 11, 24, 41

lithium 57, 58

liver 2, 3, 13, 23, 24, 30, 64, 86, 87, 112, 133, 171, 174, 179, 180, 182, 185, 186, 190, 191, 197, 213, 214

detoxification, Phase I 134, 181, 182, 183, 185

detoxification, Phase II 134, 182, 184, 185

longevity 10, 119, 165

Lou Gehrig's Disease. See ALS

Lundberg Farms 111

lung 2, 3, 31, 64, 71, 79, 112, 116, 125, 130, 138, 170, 214, 221

lutein 16, 128, 130

lycopene 128, 130

M

ma huang 136, 171, 195

Macrobiotic diet 159, 160, 162, 165, 226

macrophages 50

macular degeneration 23, 31, 130

magnesium 10, 11, 17, 18, 21, 22, 41, 57, 58, 75, 93, 146, 148, 163, 182, 207

Make A Wish Foundation 67

malignant 86

malnutrition 9, 18, 42

maltose 34, 39

manganese 11, 12, 16, 17, 18, 21, 22, 24, 41, 57, 58, 176, 214

marijuana vi, 56, 162

Marshall, Dr. Barry 82

Masai tribe 83

massage 153, 203

Mayo Clinic 107

McDonald, Evy 65, 227

meat 12, 29, 31, 48, 49, 93, 129, 146, 162, 169, 175, 187, 208

medications 173

meditation 27, 144, 155, 156

melatonin 90, 214

About the Author

Dr. Elizabeth Walker started her health career in 1974 as a dental hygienist. It was during that time she became exposed to natural forms of healing such as chiropractic and nutrition. Because the condition of the teeth and gums reflects the health of the entire body, she became fascinated by how quickly health problems could be improved by changing diet, nutrition and oral hygiene habits.

In 1982, she graduated with honors from the National College of Chiropractic in Lombard, Illinois, with a B.S. degree in Human Biology, a certificate in Acupuncture and Meridian therapy, and a Doctor of Chiropractic degree.

From 1983 to 1985 she taught physiotherapy and was a part-time clinician at Cleveland Chiropractic College in Kansas City, Missouri. She also was a test writer for two years in the subject of physiotherapy for the National Board of Chiropractic Examiners.

From 1982 to 1998, she practiced in Kansas City, Missouri. She began speaking and writing during that time as a means to educate and inform the public on wellness, regeneration and disease prevention. During her career she has attended hundreds of hours of post-graduate seminars in chiropractic, nutrition, Functional Medicine, Macrobiotics and Oriental Medicine. Since 1999, she has practiced in Fort Collins, Colorado.

CONQUER FATIGUE FUND RAISERS

This book is available for fund raising projects as a healthy alternative to the traditional candy and cookie sales. Dr. Walker will donate $5 per book to sport clubs, churches, schools, non-profit organizations, as well as individuals who are suffering from a devastating illness.

Please send an inquiry explaining the purpose of the fund-raiser and how many people will be involved to:

Vitality Doctor, 1700 South College Avenue, Suite C, Fort Collins, CO 80525

Or: **drwalker@conquerfatigue.com**

Resolve to Get Healthier!

Check Your Local Bookstore, Online Book Seller
or Place Your Order Here

Please send me the following items:

Quantity*	Title	Unit Price	Total
_____	*Conquer Fatigue in 30 Days*	$ 19.95	$ _____

Sales Tax (CO Only) $_____

†Foreign Shipping and Overnight Orders:
Call for a price quote at 970-224-0774

Shipping & Handling ($6.95)† $_____

Total Order $_____

Checks/Money Orders Payable to:
Vitality Doctor

# Books	Cost	Tax (CO Only)
1 Book	$19.95	$1.34
2 Books	$39.90	$2.67
3 Books	$59.85	$4.01
4 Books	$79.80	$5.35
5 Books	$99.75	$6.68
6 Books	$119.70	$8.02

*Contact us for Quantity Discounts!

By Phone: Toll-free (888) 764-2151 or (970) 224-0774
By Fax: (970) 224-0783
By Email: drwalker@conquerfatigue.com
On-line: www.conquerfatigue.com
By Mail: Fill out the information below and send with your remittance to:
Vitality Doctor
1700 South College Avenue, Suite C
Fort Collins, CO 80525 USA

Please Print:

Name_____Organization_____

Billing Address_____

Shipping Address_____

City/State/Postal Code _____

Country_____Phone_____Email_____

Master Card / Visa / Discover #_____Exp. Date_____

Signature _____

**For Information on using *Conquer Fatigue in 30 Days* as a fund-raiser
please contact us by email, phone, or mail!**